A Functional Approach to Group Work in Occupational Therapy

Third Edition

A Functional Approach to Group Work in Occupational Therapy

Margot C. Howe, EdD, OTR, FAOTA
Professor Emeritus
Tufts University–Boston School of Occupational Therapy
Medford, Massachusetts

Sharan L. Schwartzberg, EdD, OTR, FAOTA
Professor and Chair
Tufts University–Boston School of Occupational Therapy
Medford, Massachusetts

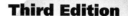 LIPPINCOTT WILLIAMS & WILKINS
A **Wolters Kluwer** Company
Philadelphia · Baltimore · New York · London
Buenos Aires · Hong Kong · Sydney · Tokyo

Editor: John Butler
Managing Editor: Ulita Lushnycky
Marketing Manager: Debby Hartman
Production Editor: Lisa JC Franko

351 West Camden Street
Baltimore, Maryland 21201-2436 USA

530 Walnut Street
Philadelphia, Pennsylvania 19106 USA

Printed in the United States of America

Library of Congress Cataloging-in-Publication Data

Howe, Margot C.
    A functional approach to group work in occupational therapy / Margot C. Howe, Sharan L. Schwartzberg.—3rd ed.
      p. cm.
    Includes bibliographical references and index.
    ISBN 0-7817-2109-1
    1. Occupational therapy. 2. Group psychotherapy. I. Schwartzberg, Sharan L. II. Title.

RM735 .H68 2001
615.8'515—dc21   00-053505

To purchase additional copies of this book call our customer service department at (800) 638-3030 or fax orders to (301) 824-7390. International customers should call (301) 714-2324.

01 02 03
1 2 3 4 5 6 7 8 9 10

To our students,
whose interest and response inspired
our continued study of group work.

Foreword

Relation is mutual. My Thou affects me, as I affect it. We are moulded by our pupils and built up by our works. (BUBER, 1958, P. 15)

... Every social organism must attend to four major tasks to keep existing. It must acquire resources from the environment to keep the members of the group alive: a hunting group must find game, a university must find students, a bank has to find deposits. Second, it must coordinate its activities with those of other groups in the pursuit of its goals. Third, it must divide the resources and the tasks within the group while maintaining harmony and cooperation among members of the group. And finally, it must develop and maintain values and beliefs that give the group hope, identity, and purpose. (CSIKSZENTMIHALYI, 1993, P. 286)

Recently my dentist asked me, "What do occupational therapists do?" I answered that occupational therapists employ purposeful activity to develop people's skills so that they can function in their daily lives in the presence of or possibility of developing *any* disability that might interfere with their competence, throughout the entire life span. (Notice that I left out the fact that we work with both individuals and groups.) He looked at me incredulously. "How can you possibly prepare students to do that?" he asked. "That has been the greatest challenge of my life as an educator," I replied. "Occupational therapists must learn to deal with human complexity because of the very nature of people and their activities."

This book represents a pioneering effort to educate occupational therapists for a complex and sophisticated subject: the knowledge, skills, and values required to develop functional groups so that individuals may learn how to better fulfill their roles as members of social systems. The authors note that they decided to write this book because of the paucity of educational material available on how to teach group process. The lack was not just in the area of group process but, more significantly, group process as seen through the unique lenses of two occupational therapists.

The emphasis in *A Functional Approach to Group Work in Occupational Therapy* is not "talk groups" or cathartic psychotherapy groups but rather how occupations may be used to develop the rules, habits, and skills required for successful living in a social environment. Engagement in activity in a group context becomes the means to the end of enabling people to achieve their goals and intentions more fully.

The lenses of the authors reflect the "optimistic vote of confidence in human nature," which Reilly (1962) believed to be an essential component of occupational therapy. Rather than focusing on diagnosis and pathology, this book emphasizes the "reservoir of sensitivity and skill" that resides in every human being and that "can be tapped" for health (Reilly, 1962), in this case, through the use of groups engaged in occupation.

In its philosophy and practice, this book promotes a different view of health than that embedded in the traditional disease model. Health, rather than being an absence of disease or pathology, is seen instead as possession of a repertoire of skills by which people can achieve their own intentions, goals, and purposes. The authors' view of health is compatible with occupational therapy's traditional concern for people who have chronic conditions. It provides a great deal of hope for people who may never be "normal" according to medical criteria.

In the current millennium, societies around the globe will be struggling with the issue of how to integrate people with disabilities into the daily routines that provide them with a place in their culture (Beisser, 1989). Occupational therapists often act as a bridge between the world of medicine and the real world of family and community. This book, therefore, is on the cutting edge. The use of groups to enable people to develop new skills to meet the challenges of their environments and, in so doing, perceive themselves as competent to master those challenges, is an essential component of occupational therapy for the 21st century and beyond. Rather than the old idea that people with disabilities need to "adjust" to their "misfortune" (Bickenbach, 1993), it provides the new idea of "adaptation" or development of a goodness of fit between the individual and his or her environment. Adaptation with disability rather than adjustment to disability is emphasized. Thus it helps to restore dignity and value to people with disability and places them, appropriately, within the mainstream of humanity.

This book is both intellectually challenging and practical. It provides stimulating, generative ideas by presenting a new model of practice, called a Model of Group Work, complete with a set of explicit assumptions, comprehensive principles, concepts, and strategies. The model retains the necessary complexity required to explain how people engaged in occupation together can "influence the state of their own health" (Reilly, 1962). The work is unique in presenting case studies that illustrate the occupational therapists' actions and thought process during the evolution of two different kinds of groups, including an honest explanation of problems arising and successes achieved.

Finally, this work contributes to a holistic, nonreductionist, generalist perception of the occupational therapist's scope of practice. In this era of specialism, it is refreshing and inspiring to read about a model of practice that puts the human being back together again and is concerned with his or her ability to function effectively, with others, in the real world.

Elizabeth J. Yerxa
Bishop, California

References

Beisser, A. (1989). Flying Without Wings: Personal Reflections on Being Disabled. New York: Doubleday.

Bickenbach, J. E. (1993). Physical Disability and Social Policy. Toronto: University of Toronto Press.

Buber, M. (1958). I and Thou (2nd ed.). New York: Charles Scribner's Sons.

Csikszentmihalyi, M. (1993). The Evolving Self: A Psychology for the Third Millennium New York: Harper Collins.

Reilly, M. (1962). Occupational therapy can be one of the great ideas of 20th century medicine. American Journal of Occupational Therapy, 16: 300–308.

Preface

Groups are a part of people's experience not only in normal or healthy life but also in life interrupted by disease and distress. Because of the potential benefits of group work and its versatility, a variety of professionals use this format in settings as diverse as hospitals, schools, businesses, and governmental agencies.

Many books have been written about group process, but most have been directed toward psychotherapy, social case work, or organizational development. Until the time of the publication of the first edition of this book, none addressed the unique orientation of occupational therapy group work that is skills-oriented, action-oriented, and here-and-now-oriented. As occupational therapy educators, we had to rely on material developed by other disciplines. We were concerned with the limitations and biases that this may have brought to our profession's practice and education.

In writing this book it is our goal to present a model for group work—a functional approach to group work—that combines theory, research, and practice in occupational therapy. Rather than being derived from other frames of reference in occupational therapy, it is a model of practice in its own right. Because the model is based on our experience and practice in teaching and conducting occupational therapy groups, as well as our research in group work, this book is presented from the vantage points of the normal group, the therapeutic group, and the occupational focus group, or functional group.

It is important for a model to be expanded and evaluated through research and the empirical evidence of clinical practice because this is how the validity of a model is tested. We are encouraged that this third edition can feature research studies that verify aspects of the theoretical model. These have been conducted since the inception of the functional group model. Other studies relating to issues of group intervention in occupational therapy are also presented and discussed.

The material in this book is organized to lead the reader through the logic of planning, implementing, and evaluating a functional group. The content is not focused on a verbal, insight-oriented approach to group work; rather, we explain the functional group as a method to aid individuals in adaptation to their life roles and tasks through occupation, the "doing" or "action," in a group. The model we propose is an approach designed for people with physical, social, emotional, or developmental problems, as well as those desirous of maintaining health and well-being. It is an approach that stems primarily from occupational therapy philosophy and practice. We offer you insights from our fruitful professional collaboration and friendship for more than 20 years.

Margot C. Howe, EdD, OTR, FAOTA
Mount Shasta, California

Sharan L. Schwartzberg, EdD, OTR, FAOTA
Boston, Massachusetts
July 2000

Acknowledgments

A book such as *A Functional Approach to Group Work in Occupational Therapy* is not conceptualized or completed without contributions from many people. We wish to thank Anne Briggs and Linda Duncombe for their help in the very initial stages of the book and Linda's continuing research on the material in Chapter 3 for edition 2; Virginia Drachman, Paul Nash, and Kathlyn Reed for their welcome expertise in model development and historical analysis; the Tufts University–Boston School of Occupational Therapy for the use of their photographs; Glenda Wong Jeong for her assistance in drawing; and Ann Bonner for her patience and skill in managing department-related activities so that scholarship could be pursued. We also wish to acknowledge the financial support that initially allowed us to research and develop a model for occupational therapy group work: Everest and Jennings, S & S Arts and Crafts, Roylan Medical Products, and the Mabel Louise Riley Research Fund of Tufts University–Boston School of Occupational Therapy.

For the third edition, there are more people we wish to thank in joining our efforts. Our gratitude to the settings and to Mary Barnes, Jennifer Berry and the Tufts University–Boston School of Occupational Therapy group practicum students for the current functional group work photos; to Mark Morelli and Edie Wieder for the class photo; and to Sarah Brezinsky our photographer for her energy and insight into group process and occupational therapy. Finally, we forever thank Nancy Keebler for her superb editorial assistance in enhancing the book's appearance and content as well as enthusiasm for the work; to our reviewers and editors and staff at Lippincott Williams & Wilkins, Margaret Biblis, Ulita Lushnycky, and Amy Amico for seeing that the tradition of group work in occupational therapy is brought into the 21st Century.

Contents

Part III
Teaching and Research

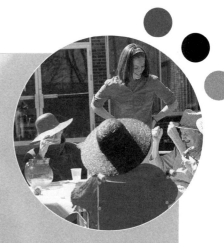

Part I
Group Work and the Functional Group Model

The recognition of group work in occupational therapy is a relatively recent development, and the use of groups as a modality is increasing in many areas of practice. Although the importance of constructive activity in maintaining and recovering the health of individuals has been acknowledged for centuries, only in recent times have practitioners and researchers attempted a systematic approach to the use of group work as a therapeutic procedure. In this section of the book, the authors will offer a historical perspective of group work in occupational therapy. From its inception, the profession of occupational therapy has developed gradually on the premise of occupation as a method of practice, not a goal (Nelson, 1997). Similarly, the practice of group occupational therapy has evolved with the times, the culture, and the experiences and observations of the therapists, to the consequent benefits of the group participants. Through learning from our experiences as practitioners and

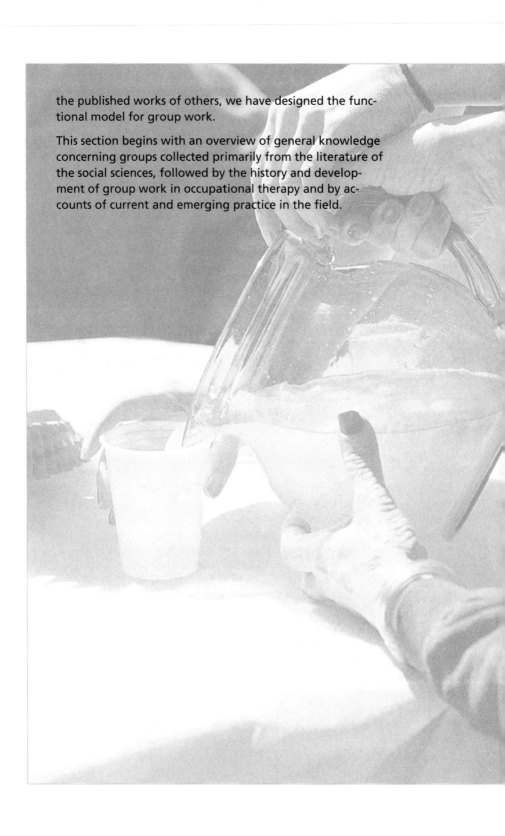

the published works of others, we have designed the functional model for group work.

This section begins with an overview of general knowledge concerning groups collected primarily from the literature of the social sciences, followed by the history and development of group work in occupational therapy and by accounts of current and emerging practice in the field.

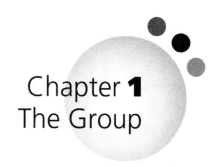

Chapter 1
The Group

Every group develops its own unique character, yet all groups present to the observer certain common features that enable us to speak of the dynamics of groups. (BENJAMIN, 1978, P. 6)

Group life has always played an important role in civilization, and throughout history, people have considered groups to be essential to survival. We are born into a family group and later expand our social network to include work groups, social groups, recreational groups, and the like. Through groups, we avoid isolation and learn about ourselves and other people. Many of us participate in group processes even when we are unaware of doing so.

The knowledge we have about groups and how they function is the result of social science research conducted during the last 60 years. Studies in group dynamics have led to a clear definition of the characteristics of groups and thus have increased our understanding of a group's potential for bringing about change in organizational behavior and for achieving therapeutic and educational goals. In this chapter, we define the concept of a group and discuss the various characteristics of groups. We also briefly describe the properties that make a group therapeutic. Finally, we present an overview of four models of group treatment.

Definition of a Group

There are many possible definitions of a group. Mosey (1973) offers the most basic definition: "A group is an aggregate of people who share a common purpose which can be attained only by group members interacting and working together" (p. 45). According to Shaefer, Johnson, and Wherry (1982), "A therapeutic group can be defined as a small, face-to-face group designed to produce behavior change in its members" (p. 2). Mosey's definition is broader and more relevant to this book because it does not exclude groups that may be involved in an activity that precludes meeting face to face on an ongoing basis. Loeser (1957) defined a group by describing some of its major characteristics:

- Dynamic interaction among members. The group process is diminished when most of the action takes place between the individual member and the leader.
- A common goal. The absence of a common goal diminishes group functioning; a shared, clear goal facilitates group functioning.
- A dependence on a proper relationship between size and function. When groups are either too large or too small, they cannot function effectively.
- A dependence on volition and consent. A group functions well only when its members consent freely to be part of that group.
- A capacity for self-determination. The group functions best in a democratic climate.

We can better grasp these characteristics if we examine a concrete example. Consider a group of people going home from work on a bus. Each of Loeser's characteristics (Box 1-1) could possibly be applied except for the group's lack of a

---

Box 1-1
Group Characteristics

Major characteristics of a group, as defined by Loeser, (1957) are:

- Dynamic interaction among members
- A common goal
- A dependence on a proper relationship between size and function
- A dependence on volition and consent
- A capacity for self-determination

common goal and self-determination. Even though the riders are aware of other people around them, they are reacting to the bus ride on an individual basis. As long as this is so, they are more accurately called an aggregate or a crowd rather than a group. They would not be called a group until they had an awareness of their dependence on each other to accomplish a goal and an acceptance of the need to interact and meet together to achieve that goal.

Two other qualities of groups are included in Hulda Knowles and Malcolm Knowles' (1959) definition of a group. These are (1) a "group consciousness—the members think of themselves as a group, have a 'collective perception of unity,' a conscious identification with each other" (p. 39), and (2) the "ability to act in a unitary manner—the group can behave as a single organism" (p. 40). These two features characterize a mature group, one that has worked together for some time to achieve cohesion.

Social scientists have attempted to classify groups according to common characteristics. Cooley (1909), a sociologist, recognized the special role of the family in the development of young children. He viewed the contacts that occurred within the family as typical of a primary group. A primary group includes close, face-to-face relationships; this type of contact is found in the family, children's play groups, and neighborhood groups. Relationships between people in primary groups are characterized by a sense of interdependence and belonging rather than a sense of individualism. A sense of "we" rather than a sense of "I" prevails in these groups. Primary groups remain an important source of nurturing and support for adults. Primary group relationships for adults are found in groups of close friends and in small, informal work groups where the emphasis is on closeness, informality, and satisfaction of personal needs. In contrast to the primary group, the secondary group is characterized by a more formal relationship between members. Secondary groups may also be small, face-to-face groups, but relations are less intimate than in primary groups. Professional groups, in which people relate more formally through their work roles, are examples of secondary groups. The relationships are work-related or task-related, entailing a more reasoned, less private interpersonal style (Box 1-2).

Box 1-2
Distinguishing Features

Social scientists such as Cooley (1909) described groups by their common traits:

Primary group: A group distinguished by close, face-to-face relationships like those found in the family, children's play groups and neighborhood groups

Secondary group: A group in which relationships are less personal, such as professional groups that focus primarily on work or tasks

In reality, the distinction between primary and secondary, formal and informal groups is not as clear cut as in Cooley's description. For instance, although a work group may maintain impersonal and formal relations between workers on the job so that they can get their work done, at the same time the group may be sincerely concerned with the members' feelings about one another. Thus the group combines the features of both primary and secondary groups. The two types of group behavior may be viewed as functions that are present in all groups but in varying proportions (Box 1-3). Benne and Sheats (1978) described these functions as (1) group task functions, which enable the group to get its work done and to achieve its goals; and (2) group-building and maintenance functions, which contribute to the building of relationships and cohesiveness among group members.

Two features are common to all groups: content and process. *Content* refers to the work done during the time that the group meets. This includes what is said and discussed, both verbally and nonverbally. *Process* refers to how things are said and done and how the group's goals are accomplished. These two features appear in every group—be it a meeting of the board of directors or a gathering of friends.

These general features or characteristics of a group are common to all groups and appear in numerous definitions presented by social scientists. Beyond these broad features, each group exists as an individual entity and is unlike any other group. As we look closely at different sorts of groups, we shall find various combinations of characteristics that define the specific groups more precisely. The specific characteristics we shall examine are structure, context and climate, composition, cohesion, and stages of development.

Characteristics of Groups

Group Structure

The structure of a group can be defined as the group form, the combination of mutually connected and dependent parts of a group (Howe, 1968a, 1968b). All groups have structure. When we look at group structure, we look

---

Box 1-3
Group Behavior

The types of behaviors that all groups exhibit were divided into two types by Benne and Sheats (1978):

Group task functions enable the group to complete its work and achieve its goals.

Groups building and maintenance functions help members build relationships and cohesiveness.

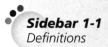

Sidebar 1-1
Definitions

Features common to all groups:
- **Content:** What members say to each other
- **Process:** The ways in which things are said; how the work of the group is carried out

at the organization and procedures of the group, considering not only what type of structure the group exhibits but also how much or how little structure is present. These factors will influence the capacity of a group to reach its goals. For instance, when a group that conducts its business according to *Robert's Rules of Order* is compared with a group that makes decisions through an informal decision-making process, it is easy to see that the two groups exhibit different structures. In the first group, all communication between members is channeled through the chairperson, and decisions are made by a majority vote. In the second group, all communication occurs directly between members without the intervention of a leader. In the latter case, the group may be more spontaneous, but it may also be less efficient. If we look still more closely, we find that although the decision-making process may take a longer time to complete, the results may give members greater satisfaction. Group structure is created from a number of factors, such as the nature of the specific goals of the group, the pattern of leader and member interaction, the composition of membership, the history of the group, and the group climate (Fig. 1-1).

Group Context and Climate

No group exists in a vacuum; rather, it exists in a historical and environmental context. A group may exist because of a historical precedent, and this may be openly stated. A hospital administrator may say, "We've always had an exercise group for our stroke patients." Or a group may be formed in response to a recognized need, such as the need for patients to discuss their plans before leaving the hospital. Still another example of a historical context would be the attitudes that surrounded the formation of a new group. A group that had been the focus of staff controversy in its planning stages may develop an attitude of suspicion toward curious nonmembers. In each of these examples, the historical context is a unique factor influencing the structure of the group. This context may make it difficult for the group to restate or alter its goals, broaden or redefine its membership roles, or refocus its activities. The prestige or attractiveness of the group for its members may also be related to the historical context. A newly organized group is often believed to

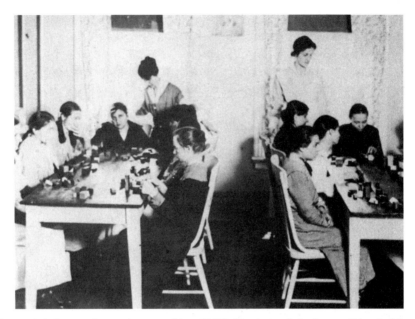

Figure 1-1. Face-to-face task groups (circa 1935). (Courtesy of the Boston School of Occupational Therapy Archives, Tufts University, Medford, MA.)

have a high prestige, thereby increasing its attractiveness for present and future members.

In contrast to historical context, which refers to the environment outside the group, the group climate refers to the physical and social environment inside the group. A physical environment that is quiet and attractive, in which members feel comfortable, is conducive to informal communication. A seating arrangement permitting face-to-face contact is essential for interpersonal communication. The physical climate is closely related to the social climate. The social climate determines whether members feel accepted, respected, or supported; the climate also determines whether the group can develop a spirit of mutuality between the leader and the members. Ideally, the group climate will be flexible so that the group can adjust to the requirements of the different group tasks.

A group can be drawn together through competition with another group. Nevertheless, many researchers question whether the attraction of mutually exclusive rewards—even in the attainment of group goals—is effective in creating an efficient environment for work (Deutsch, 1960). When people undertake a task with an attitude of cooperation and interdependence, they facilitate greater acceptance of ideas, better listening, less possessiveness of ideas, and, in general, better communication. In this type of climate, compared with one that stresses interpersonal competition, the group will strive harder to enhance its achievement and build a friendlier atmosphere.

Group Composition

Size

Group size is related not only to the goals of the group but also to the number of interactions between members. The minimum number for a group is two. Some features of a group of three are not possible in a group of two, such as members forming coalitions. In a small group, membership interaction is restricted, and the leader must initiate group action. As more members join the group, the opportunity for people to interact with a variety of individuals increases. If one of the goals of the group is to get feedback and consensual validation for member behavior, the group must be large enough to ensure a variety of opinions. Beyond a certain size, the opportunity that each member has to interact with other group members decreases. Frequently, in large groups, only the most assertive members of the group are able to express themselves.

The question of group size has been studied extensively by group dynamics researchers. Bales and Borgatta (1962) observed task groups of two to seven members and found that group size influenced communication patterns. Groups with an even number of members (four or six) had significantly more disagreements and antagonisms and less expression of positive feelings than did groups with an odd number of members (three, five, or seven). Asch (1960) studied small groups and investigated the effect that the size of the majority has on group pressure. He found that a majority of four or more did not produce effects greater than did a smaller majority of three. The main change in group pressure occurred when the majority changed from two to three members. Castore (1962) studied the effects of group size on the number of member-to-member interactions in therapy groups and found that there was a substantial reduction in the number of interactions when the group size reached nine or more members. Similarly, Hare (1962) noted that larger groups produce lower member satisfaction and that as the size of a group increases, the time available for each member to participate decreases.

Open or closed groups

The membership in an open group frequently changes from one group session to the next. A continuous turnover in membership occurs as some people leave the group and others join it (Box 1-4). In an open group, a significant time and effort is devoted to introducing new members to the group. Because each group of individuals develops a unique climate, the introduction of new members changes the climate and alters member security. Hare (1962) found in his studies of small groups that the rate of member turnover in open groups influenced group cohesiveness.

Groups in which the membership remains constant are called closed groups. Cohesiveness and trust are maximized in closed groups, and thus the potential for learning and behavior change is increased. Yalom (1983) found that cohesiveness and a stable membership are not always constructive. He suggests that over time closed groups might profit from a change in membership.

> Box 1-4
> **Group Structure**
>
> Open group: A group where the membership may change from session to session.
>
> Closed group: A group where the membership stays the same for the duration of the group and no new members can be added.

Members in some of the groups he studied stated that the experience of seeing members leave the group increased the pressure on them to do something for themselves. New members also provided old members with an opportunity to help others and practice social skills with strangers.

The length of time over which a group meets is probably not as important as the total number of hours or sessions. For instance, a group may meet three times per week for three weeks or once per week for nine weeks. The total number of hours will be the same. The more frequent sessions, however, may increase the intensity of the group experience for the members. In the last few years, social scientists have experimented with varying lengths of group time. Marathon groups or extended time sessions over weekends have become popular. Under the pressure of time, the development of the group is accelerated and members undergo a more intense experience. Another factor that determines the length of the group meeting is the time needed for the group to process. Longer processing frequently happens with certain group populations, for example, the elderly or individuals who are depressed or confused. It is not unusual for the length of time that a group meets to be determined by internal factors, such as the time required to complete the chosen task. We often hear of this group as the task force appointed to investigate a specific problem. In other groups, the length may be determined by the time required to meet the group goals. In schools, groups are commonly timed according to external factors such as the length of a semester or a school year.

Voluntary or involuntary membership
Group members come together for many reasons, and the motives of the individual members can affect the success of a group in achieving its goals (Box 1-5). Although members may share a common concern, whether or not members joined the group of their own volition can affect the functioning of the group. Involuntary membership may result in apathy or rebellion. The relative attractiveness of members to a group will determine the degree of cohesiveness of that group.

In their research, Cartwright and Zander (1960) identified two factors that attracted members to a group: (1) the group itself was viewed as a desirable object, and (2) group membership was viewed as a way to satisfy needs that existed outside the group. A group could be deemed attractive because of the activities available in the group, because of the people who constituted its

> **Box 1-5**
> **Concurrent Goals**
>
> Personal goals: Group members may be working toward individual goals.
> Group goals: The group aims for its own set of goals.

membership, or both. For instance, a cooking group may be attractive to members because they like to cook and eat the results of their work. On the other hand, the cooking group may be attractive to members because they want to be with people who are members of that group. They may not be interested in cooking at all. Group behavior is frequently influenced by the degree to which membership in the group is a result of personal choice or compulsion.

Evidence from research suggests that if people are attracted to membership, they are more likely to accept the responsibilities of membership (Dion, Miller, and Magnan, 1970). They will also attend the meetings with more regularity (Back, 1951) and persevere in achieving difficult goals (Horwitz, 1960). Members attracted to the group place greater value on the group goals than do members who are not attracted or who are forced to attend (Zander and Havelin, 1960). This research supports the view that benefits are greater from voluntary membership than from involuntary membership. This does not mean that all compulsory membership is unattractive. All people are members of involuntary groups such as the family group, racial groups, and classroom groups. Groups in which membership is not a matter of choice can lead to satisfaction and growth. Lifton (1961) aptly noted that membership in involuntary groups can be a source of security, particularly for dependent individuals.

Group goals

The goals for a group may be specific or general. Either someone outside the group or the group itself can determine these goals. How a group is formed and who holds authority for the group may dictate whether goals can be changed and by whom they can be changed. Authorities other than the group leader often specify and regulate the goals of the group. For example, the administrator of a nursing home organizes a group of patients to make decorations for a social event, and the occupational therapy assistant is assigned to lead the group. In this case, the administrator, who is not part of the group, determines the group task and goals, not the group itself or even the group leader.

A group may have more than one goal. Group goals can be a composite of the goals of individual members or a product of the group, the development of the goals representing an effort shared by all members.

Frequently, two levels of goals coexist: personal goals and group goals (Box 1-6). While the group is working toward one common goal, members may also be working toward individual goals. When these two levels are compatible, the group will function effectively to reach its goals. When these two levels are incompatible, the goals will need to be reexamined and modified. Similarly, the group leader may have one set of goals and the membership another set of goals. These two sets of goals may be compatible or in conflict with each other. How the various goals are related will influence the achievement of both sets of goals.

Groups fare better when members are clear about their goals. Raven and Rietsema (1957) studied the effect of clarity of goals on the member roles. Group members who had a clear understanding of the goals experienced greater feelings of group belongingness and were more involved in the process of achieving those goals. The more time a group spent in working out agreement on clear objectives, the faster it could reach those goals, and the more likely it was that members would reach a consensus. Cartwright and Zander (1960) found that when all members of the group accepted a single goal, they became interdependent and were able to improve the quality of group performance through a process of mutual facilitation.

As a group works together to determine its goals, integrate personal goals into group goals, and reevaluate the goals and perhaps change them, it increases its productivity. Through working together, group members increase their knowledge of one another and of how they can best work together (Box 1-7). Lippitt (1961) outlined four steps that enable a group to increase its productivity:

Box 1-7
Group Productivity

To increase its productivity (Lippitt, 1961), a group should:

- Have at the outset a clear understanding of the goals it wants to reach.
- Be aware of its own process, continually evaluate that process and make necessary changes.
- Be aware of and understand the skills, talents, and other resources within its membership.
- Create new tasks as needed and terminate those tasks no longer compatible with the goals.

1. A group should have at the outset a clear understanding of the goals it wants to reach.
2. The group should be aware of its own process. It should continually evaluate that process and make necessary changes.
3. The group should be aware of and understand the skills, talents, and other resources within its membership.
4. The group should create new tasks as needed and terminate those tasks no longer compatible with the goals.

Groups need to choose goals that they can reach within the limitations of their resources. Groups that are realistic about their aspirations are successful in reaching goals, according to Atkinson and Feather (1966). Also, when a group is given a set of alternatives, the group will select a higher risk alternative than will an individual member (Bem, Wallach, and Kogan, 1965).

Leader and membership interaction

The pattern of interaction and communication among all group members can differ from group to group. This interaction can be predominantly verbal, as in group therapy sessions, or mainly physical or active, as in a cooking group preparing a meal. The interactional pattern may be highly structured or informal, spontaneous, and loosely structured. An example of a structured interactional pattern is the high-level inpatient therapy group described by Yalom (1983). In this therapy group, he introduced a structure called an agenda go-round; according to this structure, each member formulated a personal agenda for the group session and shared his or her goals for the session with the group. This structure assured that all members would speak up in the meeting and talk about their personal goals in therapy. This can be contrasted with an informal, loosely structured group in which members may or may not talk as they choose. When they do interact, they choose the context of their own interactions (Box 1 8).

The nature of the group goals and the type of activity will influence the interactional pattern. Consider a group whose task is to prepare a meal. The planning phase will be mainly verbal. After this phase has been completed, members will work individually or in dyads while the meal is being prepared. The group interactional pattern must change if the task is to be completed effectively.

Box 1-8
Interactional Patterns

A high-level inpatient therapy group is an example of a structured interactional pattern (Yalom, 1983). Group members took part in an agenda go-round in which participants came up with a personal agenda for the session and shared their goals for that session. In this format, all members spoke up and discussed their personal goals.

The studies of Lewin, Lippitt, and White (1939) on the impact of different leadership styles on group behavior have shown that leadership influences the group interactional pattern. Under autocratic leadership, the interaction of members was found to be formal and hostile. When the leader assumed a democratic style, the interaction patterns of the members were more informal and cooperative. This study will be discussed in more detail in Chapter 5.

A number of different factors influence communication patterns in groups. Festinger and Thibaut (1951) found that between 70% and 90% of the communication in the groups that they studied was addressed to persons whose opinions were at the extremes of the existing range of group opinions. Hurwitz, Zander, and Hymovitch (1960) determined that members with "low power" in the group spoke up less and were more conspicuous in their behavior than "high-power" members. Further, low-power members were less liked by both high-power and low-power members. In this study, the term *high-power members* referred to persons who had been evaluated as having prestige and the ability to persuade others.

The rules and regulations of membership may also influence the group interactional pattern. Rules may govern attendance, participation, types of acceptable behavior, or the assignment of duties or roles. In some groups, members are not allowed to leave the group before the meeting has ended; in others, they are not allowed to arrive late. The leader typically enforces these rules. Sometimes rules are agreed on by the members; then the group acts as the enforcing body.

The style of the group leader, as well as the goals of the group, will influence the roles members can assume in the group. These roles may be narrowly prescribed, or they may be varied, leaving members free to assume different roles as the need arises. According to Benne and Sheats (1978), roles for group members are of three kinds. First is the "group task role"; its purpose is to assist the group in coordinating its efforts to define and solve common problems. Second is the "group building and maintenance role," which helps the group to function as a group. Members in this role focus on the processes developed to enable everyone to work together as a group and on strengthening or altering those processes as needed. Third is the "individual role," which is concerned solely with the satisfaction of individual needs. Benne and Sheats (1978) have described member roles within each of these types.

Twelve roles can be classified as group task roles that assist the work of the group in completing specified task goals (Box 1-9).

- The *initiator–contributor* suggests or proposes new ideas or new ways of viewing the group problems or goals.
- The *information seeker* asks for clarification of suggestions made and for authoritative information and facts pertinent to the problem being discussed.
- The *opinion seeker* asks not primarily for the facts of the case but for clarification of the values pertinent to what the group is doing.
- The *information giver* offers facts or generalizations that are authoritative or relates his or her own experiences to the group problem.

> ## Box 1-9
> ### Group Task Roles
>
> Group task roles help a group complete specified task goals (Benne and Sheats, 1978). These roles are:
>
> - Initiator-contributor
> - Information seeker
> - Opinion seeker
> - Information giver
> - Opinion giver
> - Elaborator
> - Coordinator
> - Orienter
> - Evaluator-critic
> - Energizer
> - Procedural technician
> - Recorder

- The *opinion giver* states a belief or opinion related to a suggestion made or to an alternative suggestion.
- The *elaborator* makes suggestions in terms of examples and offers a rationale for suggestions made previously.
- The *coordinator* clarifies the relationships among various ideas and suggestions, tries to pull ideas together, or tries to coordinate the activities of various members or subgroups.
- The *orienter* defines the position of the group with respect to its goals.
- The *evaluator–critic* subjects the accomplishments of the group to standards of group functioning in the context of the group task.
- The *energizer* prods the group into action or decision making and attempts to stimulate the group to a "greater" or "better" activity.
- The *procedural technician* facilitates group movement by doing things for the group.
- The *recorder* makes a record of group suggestions and decisions or writes down the products of discussion.

Group building and maintenance roles focus on building group processes and supportive attitudes and on maintaining group-centered behavior (Box 10). Seven roles comprise this category:

- The *encourager* praises, agrees with, and accepts the contributions of others. Through these attitudes, he or she indicates warmth and solidarity toward the other group members.

> Box 1-10
> **Group Maintenance Roles**
>
> Group building and maintenance roles focus on building group processes
> (Benne and Sheats, 1978). These roles are:
>
> - Encourager
> - Harmonizer
> - Compromiser
> - Gatekeeper or expediter
> - Standard setter or ego ideal
> - Group observer or commentator
> - Follower

- The *harmonizer* mediates differences between members, attempts to reconcile disagreements, and relieves tension in conflict situations.
- The *compromiser* operates from within a conflict in which his or her ideas or positions are involved. The compromiser may compromise by giving up power, admitting error, or in agreeing with the group by altering his or her opinion.
- The *gatekeeper* or *expediter* attempts to keep communication channels open by encouraging and facilitating the participation of other group members or by regulating the flow of communication in the group.
- The *standard setter* or *ego ideal* expresses standards for the group to achieve in its functioning or applies norms in evaluating the quality of the group process.
- The *group observer* or *commentator* keeps records of group process and helps the group to evaluate its own procedures by presenting feedback.
- The *follower* goes along with the sense of the group, serving as an audience in group discussion.

Individual roles are assumed by individual members of a group to satisfy personal needs that are not relevant to the group task and maintenance functions (Box 1-11). When a group experiences a high incidence of "individual-centered" rather than "group-centered" participation, the group should evaluate its functioning.

- The *aggressor* lowers the status of others; disapproves of the values, acts, and feelings of others; and attacks the whole group or an issue on which the group is working.
- The *blocker* tends to be negative, stubborn, disagreeing, and oppositional beyond reason.

> **Box 1-11**
> **Individual Roles**
>
> Some group members assume "individual-centered" roles (Benne and Sheats, 1978), such as those of:
>
> - Aggressor
> - Blocker
> - Recognition seeker
> - Self-confessor
> - Playboy
> - Dominator
> - Help seeker
> - Special interest pleader

- The *recognition seeker* works in various ways to draw attention to him or herself.
- The *self-confessor* uses the audience that the group provides to express personal, non–group-oriented communications.
- The *playboy* displays a lack of involvement in the group's processes.
- The *dominator* tries to assert personal authority or superiority by manipulating the whole group or selected members of the group. Domination may be in the form of flattery, asserting a superior status, or interrupting the contributions of others.
- The *help seeker* tries to elicit expressions of sympathy from the group through unreasonable expressions of insecurity or self-deprecation.
- The *special interest pleader* speaks for special interest groups, usually as a mask for his or her own prejudices and biases.

The interaction between the leadership and the membership of the group will determine the extent to which members can assume these different roles. Napier and Gershenfeld (1973) list some of the factors that relate to member participation in the group. According to their research, the morale of the entire group will be better in groups in which members have more access to participation: The more open the participation, the better the morale. The positions that members take in the group can influence both the leadership of the group and the potential for conflict.

The pattern of interaction between members and the leader may directly influence the problem-solving and decision-making capacity of the group. Groups commonly have problems making decisions. They frequently make a quick decision that fails when the decision is implemented, or they may be unable to reach any decision at all (Box 1-12). In both cases, inadequate discussion of the

Box 1-12
An Example of Poor Decision Making

In an afterschool group for teenagers, three or four members begin to enthusiastically plan their next group session. They discuss plans for meeting at the park. Someone says they will bring a ball. The following week, those members are very late in arriving at the group. They said, "Where were you guys? We were waiting for you at the park." The other members replied, "We didn't plan to go to the park, we never agreed to that, we thought you were just talking."

issues involved in the decision may be responsible for the lack of success. The concerns need to be brought out and discussed openly.

Sometimes, the nature or obligation of the decision is not clearly understood by the group members, and some changes need to be made. Further, members may have difficulty separating the issues from the members who proposed them. Interpersonal loyalties or conflicts may impinge on the decision-making process and outweigh the importance of the issues.

Probably the most common error in group decision making is assuming that a vote is representative of the consensus of the group. A vote is often made without the full participation of the group members; discussion leaders typically seek out members who agree with them and avoid those who have no opinion or who disagree. Lippitt (1961) compiled a list of factors that facilitate group decision making. The list includes a clearly defined problem, a defined line of responsibility, effective communication, and an appropriate group size (Box 1-13).

Box 1-13
Facilitating Factors

Factors that facilitate group decision making (Lippitt, 1961) are:

- A clear definition of the problem
- A clear understanding of who is responsible for the decision
- Effective communication for producing ideas
- An appropriate group size for decision making
- A means for testing different alternative decisions
- A commitment to the decision
- The honest commitment of the leader to the group decision-making process
- Agreement on the procedures and methods for decision making before deliberations on the issue

There are no fixed rules for good decision making, but good leadership can contribute by guiding the group along lines that support member contribution, free expression of opinions, and a unity of purpose. Rules and regulations might be unspoken or unwritten, but they are implicitly understood by members owing to factors such as prior experiences in similar groups or to previous experiences or learning.

Group Cohesiveness

The term *group cohesiveness* appears often in the literature of group dynamics and is one of the goals that groups seek to achieve. There are several definitions of the term *group cohesiveness*. All refer to the intensity of feeling that members have for the group, to their sense of solidarity, that this is "our group." The term also implies a sense of value about the group, a wish to defend the group against external and internal threats. Frank (1957) refers to this as the attractiveness that the group has for its members. Cartwright and Zander (1960) see cohesiveness as the result of all the forces acting on all the members to persuade them to remain in the group. According to Yalom (1970), "'Group cohesiveness' is not per se a curative factor but instead a pre-condition for effective therapy . . . Cohesiveness is both a determinant and effect of intermember acceptance: the members of a highly cohesive therapy group will respond to each other in this manner more frequently than members of a noncohesive group; groups with members who show high mutual understanding and acceptance are, by definition, cohesive" (p. 38).

Some of the elements that contribute to group cohesiveness are the amount of cooperation, caring, and support that exists between members; the encouragement that they show each other; group attendance rates; and member punctuality at meetings. The degree of trust and risk taking is also a measure of

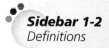

Sidebar 1-2
Definitions

Group structure: *The form or organizing procedures of the group*

Group context: *The environmental or historical setting in which the group is operating*

Group climate: *The physical and/or social environment inside a group*

Group composition: *Refers to group goals, size, membership, format*

Group cohesiveness: *The intensity of positive feelings that members have for the group and their sense of belonging to the group*

Group goals: *What the group is seeking to accomplish*

Interactional pattern: *How members interact in the group, for example, who talks to whom*

cohesiveness, as is the amount of group support given to individual members who express their opinions and share their points of view.

Stages of Group Development

Just as the individuals who compose them, groups pass through several stages or phases of development during their existence. These phases have been labeled in various ways according to the behavioral theories held by the observers. In the beginning stages of a group, the members need to get to know each other and to develop a sense of being comfortable in the group. After the group has been meeting for a period, members develop ways of interrelating and working together. The path of development is not a straight line, and frequently groups revert to a previous developmental stage when there is a change in structure or the group is under stress.

Bion (1959), a researcher who contributed extensively to the field of group dynamics from a psychoanalytic point of view, focused on the tensions experienced by group members and the resolution of these tensions in the process of group development. Group members coped with their tensions in three stages: (1) through fighting or fleeing, (2) through dependence and counterdependence on the leader, and (3) through a process of pairing. Bion (1959) concluded that the pairing of the third stage was a way of creating closer bonds between members and thus overcoming the underlying fears and tensions.

William Schutz (1960) presented a theory of group development based on interpersonal needs. He described three stages: inclusion, control, and affection. The inclusion stage involved issues related to belonging or not belonging to the group; the control stage involved issues of dependence and authority; and the affection stage involved issues of intimacy, closeness, and caring.

Bales (1955 a,b) and Tuckman (1965) also investigated the dynamics of small groups and described similar stages of group development (Box 1-14). Tuckman (1965) labeled and outlined four stages. In the first stage, all groups have to deal with the issues of coming together and forming a group. They need to get to know each other, their resources and talents, and their tasks. The second stage is a time of conflict, with disagreement concerning the task and how

---

Box 1-14
Developmental Stages

The four stages of group development (Tuckman, 1965) are:

- Forming
- Storming
- Norming
- Performing

it should be completed. Conflicts may also arise regarding group leadership. By the third stage, the conflicts have been resolved, and the group can develop norms and procedures to carry out its activities. In the final stage, a cohesive unit has begun to form. The group is in control and can work effectively on the task at hand.

According to Tuckman's (1965) model of group development, the conflicts of the storming stage are a normal event in the development of a group.

Bennis and Shepard (1956) present yet another theory of group development based on their studies of group dynamics. Before outlining their stages of development, they delineate two major areas of uncertainty for group members: (1) orientation to authority and power and (2) orientation toward each other. The first phase of this developmental model is concerned with dependence and power relations and includes three subphases. Subphase one, dependence-flight, refers to member behavior designed to please the leader in the hope that the leader will ease the member's anxiety and find a goal and task for him or her. Trying to be polite, members engage in "flight" behavior because they discuss matters external to the group. As the leader continues to "fail" the group by not making decisions for the members, expressions of counterdependence replace dependence, and the group progresses to subphase two, counterdependence-fight. In this subphase, expressions of hostility are more frequent and also are supported by other members. Subgroups emerge and vie for leadership. This chaos leads to a resolution in subphase three, resolution-catharsis. During this phase, the group members assume leadership roles, and the group becomes unified in its pursuit of a goal. Pairing and involvement in the group task occurs. The subgroups fuse, and the group becomes ready to move into the second stage.

The second developmental stage of this model relates to group interdependence. In this stage, the group turns its attention to issues of shared responsibility. In subphase four, enchantment-flight, everyone is happy, and an atmosphere of "sweetness and light" prevails. Everyone is amiable and decisions are unanimous, but the decisions made are related to issues about which no one has strong feelings. The harmony of this period soon wears thin, and the group again begins to form subgroups, leading to subphase five, disenchantment. In this subphase, the group divides into subgroups based on the degree of intimacy required for membership. Again, a resolution of the problem occurs under the pressure of having to accomplish a task. The group now reaches the final subphase, consensual validation, which represents an acceptance of the group in realistic terms, with diminishing ties based on a personal orientation. Group consensus becomes easier to achieve on important issues, and personal ties develop from working together to achieve group goals.

Another group of researchers, Garland, Jones, and Kolodny (1965), who were observers with backgrounds in social group work, described five stages of group development: preaffiliation, power and control, intimacy, differentiation, and separation. Here again we see the developmental issues to be affiliation, power, intimacy, and interrelatedness or differentiation. The various reports of the research of group observers discussed earlier show remarkable agreement on the basic developmental issues of small groups.

The Group As a System

The preceding descriptions of the stages of group development are based on the processes inherent in the group as a whole, not just in members' actions or leader actions. The group is viewed as a unit, or as a system. A system is an organized body of interdependent constituent parts. It is the interactive system that changes through the developmental stages, not the individual group members. The notion of a group as a system has its origins in General Systems Theory, developed by Ludwig Von Bertalanffy (1968). A biologist, Von Bertalanffy was concerned with the manner in which living systems were organized and in how their constituent parts were interconnected and interrelated (Box 1-15).

As group workers, we are more concerned with the processes of group interaction than with the structure of the group's individual parts because the group is different from the sum of its parts. The group is more than a collection of six or seven individuals; it is composed of systems and subsystems that interact with each other and with the group as a whole.

Because the group is a living or open system it must be viewed also as the subsystem of a larger system and this is referred to as its environmental or ecological context. So, according to systems theory, the individual is seen as a sub-

---

Box 1-15
General Systems Theory

General Systems Theory was introduced by a biologist, Ludwig Von Bertalanffy in 1968. He developed the theory as an alternative to the reductionist scientific trend of the times. He believed that the way to a better understanding of living systems was not to study parts in greater detail in isolation, but rather to look at them as parts of a larger system. A system is defined as an organized unit of interdependent parts.

According to this theory, there are two basic kinds of systems: closed systems and open systems. A closed system is usually described as a mechanical system such as clockworks. An open system is descriptive of a living organism that obtains needed energy from its interaction with its environment. In an open system the boundaries between the systems and subsystems are permeable, allowing energy and information to move from one part of the system to another. This process permits the system to adjust to changing conditions as needed for continued function.

Further information on systems theory and its relevance to group work can be found in: Borg and Bruce, 1991; Bronfenbrenner, 1979; Buckley, 1968; Donigian and Malnati, 1997; and Tubbs, 1984.

system of the group, and the group is seen as the individual's environmental context. Similarly, the group is a subsystem of the organization in which it is located, and that organization comprises its environmental context. A system many be embedded in numerous layers of environments.

Complex adaptive systems such as groups are open both internally and externally. The interchange between, or among their constituent parts may result in changes in the nature of the parts themselves. The feedback process enables adaptation and self-regulation as well as self-direction. The model presented in this book in Chapter 4 presents a systems approach to group work for occupational therapy.

Therapeutic Groups

Curative Aspects of a Group

Up to this point, we have presented a basic discussion about groups; in this section, we shall turn to the aspects of groups that make them therapeutic. Researchers in group dynamics and group therapists are in ongoing disagreement regarding the nature of the therapeutic process in a group. Workers in the field of group dynamics make their observations on, and draw their conclusions from, the behavior of the group at the group level. They describe the processes originating from group interaction. By contrast, when group therapists observe similar group behavior, they typically make their observations on the individual level and see the group processes merely as an example of how individuals relate in a group setting. For group therapists, the dynamics in groups are interpersonal dynamics and therefore no different from those that occur between any two individuals. The controversy between researchers and therapists focuses on whether the group process itself has a greater impact on helping a member to change than the efforts of the therapist. Researchers have described the therapeutic factors inherent in the group, and a significant overlap and agreement among the studies are apparent (Corey and Corey, 1977; Corsini and Rosenberg, 1955; Yalom, 1975). These researchers noted that the group members described the healing processes as rooted in the interaction between the group members; rarely did the reports recognize a role played by the therapist.

Therapeutic factors in occupational therapy groups have been recently studied and compared with patients' perceptions of psychotherapy groups (Falk-Kessler, Momich, and Perel, 1991; Finn, 1989; Webster, 1988; Webster and Schwartzberg, 1992). The similarity between valued conditions across all of these groups is striking and lends further confidence to the notion that the curative nature of treatment groups is organic to the group process format. It is likely that, in addition to the three highly valued factors found in the occupational therapy groups investigated—group cohesiveness, interpersonal learning-output, and instillation of hope—there are conditions unique to occupational therapy and unlike those that are Yalom's group psychotherapy categories. Webster (1988) and Finn (1989) generated new and unique therapeutic factors in occupational therapy groups and proposed separate categories for investigation. These factors included the value of learning new skills and having an opportunity to relax and be creative. These additional factors may reflect a difference between verbal psychotherapy groups and groups used in occupational therapy intervention.

After extensive research, Yalom (1975) identified 11 factors that led to successful group therapy (Box 1-16). Many factors identified in this study were similar to those identified in other studies. Yalom's (1975) 11 curative factors are described as follows:

Instilling hope. When members are in a group with other people who are in the process of changing, their hopes are reinforced. Members in a group usually function at different points on a health continuum. Hope is nurtured when group members with similar problems appear to profit from their interactions in the group.

Universality. People who seek help in groups often feel that they are alone in their misery and that no one else could be as unacceptable as they feel they are. In the group they learn that others have similar concerns, fears, and experiences. It is reassuring for them to know that they are not truly different from other people even though they may have endured painful experiences in life.

Imparting information. Members learn a great deal about themselves and others through participation in a group. They also learn about the group process itself. Some groups provide extensive didactic information about

---

Box 1-16
Curative Factors

Yalom (1975) identified 11 factors that led to successful group therapy:

- Instilling hope
- Universality
- Imparting information
- Altruism
- Corrective recapitulation of the family group
- Development of socializing techniques
- Imitative behavior
- Catharsis
- Existential factors
- Cohesiveness
- Interpersonal learning

growth and development or about the treatment of specific diseases or states of dysfunction. Other groups teach actual skills and roles. These skills may be practiced in preparation for discharge to the home or the community.

Altruism. An important aspect of membership in a group is the opportunity to help others and to be helped by others. Members gain a feeling of self-worth when they are able to give to other members and to "make a difference" in others' lives. People need to feel that they are needed. Altruism has traditionally played an important part in the healing rites of primitive cultures.

Corrective recapitulation of the family group. The therapy group is a primary group closely resembling the family group. The leader is often perceived as a parental figure. Past familial experiences influence a member's interaction with other members and with the leader. The therapy group can help a member realize and correct maladaptive behavior that may have characterized relationships in the family group.

Development of socializing techniques. Socializing techniques, also called social learning or the learning of social skills, vary in importance and explicitness from group to group. Groups may use learning methods such as role playing and structured exercises to develop specific social skills. An example would be the use of role playing to practice applying for a job or asking someone for a date. For individuals who lack close relationships, the group may be their only opportunity for accurate interpersonal feedback that enables them to learn about another person's reactions to their standard behaviors, such as a lack of eye contact when talking or a display of indifference that may mask feelings of caring. Members in long-term groups learn how to listen, to respond to others, and to be less judgmental about themselves and others.

Imitative behavior. Group members often model their behavior on other members' behaviors. People can learn new behaviors just from watching other people. Additionally, members learn vicariously through the experience of other members who have problems similar to their own. More will be said about modeling as a method of learning in Chapter 5.

Catharsis. The expression and release of feelings are an important part of the healing process in the group. Merely expressing emotion, however, may not be of lasting benefit. Members learn to express feelings and discover that the expression of honest feelings is not as disastrous as may have been feared. People are often surprised to realize that positive and negative feelings toward a person may be present at the same time.

Existential factors. Personal concerns about isolation, death, and helplessness may be discussed and shared in the group setting. For instance, a group of people who all have a chronic disease may well discuss the limitations imposed by the disease, the areas in which they can still exercise choices, and the responsibilities they must assume for those choices. Often by facing the issues of life and death, people can live life more honestly; the group lends the support needed to face these issues.

Cohesiveness. Cohesiveness refers to the sense of group belonging and was discussed in an earlier section. Humans are social beings and need to relate to other people. For some people, isolation is a serious problem. Being hospitalized is an isolating experience for most people. The individual is separated from familial support systems, and there are few opportunities to share feelings and to be accepted on a personal level. For hospital patients in particular, the group becomes a place where sharing experiences and feelings can augment the therapeutic aspects of treatment.

Interpersonal learning. The therapy group is a microcosm of society in which persons interact in much the same way that they would in society or outside the group. By helping each other to understand their behavior within the group, members get a clearer picture of interpersonal behavior patterns in society at large. Learning in the here and now provides individuals with immediate feedback about how others see them. Thus, they learn what behavior brings people closer to them or keeps them at a distance, and on the basis of this information, they can decide whether to alter their own behavior. This is a process called "reality testing."

According to Yalom (1975), most groups include all of the 11 therapeutic factors just listed; different groups emphasize different factors. Although the curative factors are to be found within group processes and do not adhere to the role of the leader, we cannot conclude that the style and skills of the leader are of no consequence. Clearly, the leader plays an important part in helping the group members establish their interactional pattern and develop norms that assist the group to become cohesive.

Overview of Models of Group Treatment

Many types of treatment groups are conducted in a wide variety of treatment settings, but all can be described under four main categories: activity groups, intrapsychic groups, social systems groups, and growth groups. These types are not mutually exclusive; there is considerable overlap, and some groups may be a combination of two types. Tables 1-1 to 1-4 present an overview of these four models of group treatment. Each group is examined according to four factors: group goals and structure, the theoretical perspective, the role of the leader, and group membership.

Activity Groups

Group goals and structure

Activity groups are small, primary groups in which members are engaged in a common activity or task that is directed toward learning and maintaining occupational performance (Table 1-1). According to Fidler (1969):

Table 1-1
Overview of the Activity Group Treatment Model

Type of Group	Examples	Group Goal	Theoretical Perspective	Leader Role	Membership
Activity group	Evaluation, task-oriented, develop-mental, thematic, topical, and instru-mental groups	To learn and maintain occupational performance in particular regarding: 1) Task 2) Role	The role of purposeful activity ("doing") in maintaining and developing skills, a role that changes in small groups (Mosey, 1981; Fidler, 1969; Kaplan, 1988).	1) To create a group climate that facilitates interaction 2) To provide support and education 3) To structure the level of group activity	1) Hetero-geneous or homo-geneous 2) Select members according to level of skill develop-ment

The intent of the task-oriented group is to provide a shared working experience wherein the relationship between feeling, thinking and behavior, their impact on others and on task accomplishment and productivity can be viewed and explored. . . . Task accomplishment is not the purpose of the group but hopefully the means by which purpose is realized. It is seen as the catalytic agent which elicits behavior and interaction, brings into focus both functional capacities and limitations, facilitates collaboration in working through problems and provides a concrete reality factor against which to measure learning and achievement. (p. 45)

Although the goals and activities of task-oriented groups may differ, these groups have inherent structures and goals of therapeutic value for the members. With its focus on function relating to the task at hand, the activity group closely replicates living in the community or the family. In this climate, with a concrete activity on which to focus the group's attention and an opportunity for learning from direct experience, group members learn more easily and with increased understanding.

The given task provides a degree of form and organization that is helpful to many group members. When the activity goals are clear, the skills and roles necessary to meet these goals become evident, and the involvement and comfort of members increase. Members are given the opportunity to coordinate and use the skills available within the group. In this way, people can work on that part of the task in which they have greater skill. For example, a person who is shy or who has poorly developed verbal skills may become involved in the group primarily through joining in the task itself. On the other hand, a member who is afraid of the physical demands of the task or who cannot get involved because of physical limitations can participate on the verbal level. Learning occurs in the shared process of "doing," as well as through the process of discussion. In the process of doing, all available skills become important for the completion of the task, and members are drawn together in joining their skills toward accomplishing a single goal. The activity also provides a concrete measure of the progress of the group as a whole toward the achievement of the group tasks and goals. Through their individual contributions, the members may also clearly demonstrate their growth and achievement over time.

The given task of the group may serve the needs of the members in different ways. In some cases, group members may feel more comfortable working on a task than on interpersonal relationships. These members identify with the group through their involvement in the task activity. Other members may be comfortable in the group setting but have difficulty dealing with the nonhuman environment; they need the opportunity to learn how to solve specific problems through participation in a joint activity. For these members, accomplishing the task may be the major goal. For all members, a sense of belonging and partnership can result from the exploration of a shared need to master the nonhuman environment.

Mosey (1981) describes six major types of activity groups (Box 1-17). These types are not meant to be discrete, because some groups may have the properties of several categories; the description of types is meant to clarify and facilitate communication:

- *Evaluation groups:* Designed to assess an individual's areas of function and dysfunction within a group setting, thus evaluating both interpersonal and activity skills. The role of the therapist is primarily that of an observer, and the activity is chosen by the therapist.
- *Task-oriented groups:* Designed to increase members' awareness of themselves and others in the activity process and in their interactions with other members. The role of the therapist or leader is to help members explore the relationships between thoughts, feelings, and actions.
- *Developmental groups:* Designed to teach only group interaction skills, based on the theory that group interaction skills are developmentally stage

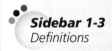

Sidebar 1-3
Definitions

Task-oriented group: *A group designed to provide a shared work experience. Learning occurs in the shared process of "doing"*

Intrapsychic group: *A group designed to focus on the processes and conflicts that occur within an individual*

> **Box 1-17**
> **Activity Groups**
>
> Mosey (1981) described six major types of activity groups. However, some groups may have the properties of several categories:
>
> - Evaluation groups
> - Task-oriented groups
> - Developmental groups
> - Thematic groups
> - Topical groups
> - Instrumental groups

specific. The role of the therapist varies with the developmental level of the group.

- *Thematic groups:* Designed to help members learn the knowledge, skills, and attitudes necessary for accomplishing a specific set of activities.
- *Topical groups:* Same goals as those of the thematic groups except that these goals are carried out independently in the community. One type of topical group, the anticipatory group, focuses on activities that the group members anticipate doing in the future. A second type of topical group, the concurrent group, focuses on activities that the group members are currently doing in the community. In this group, the therapist helps group members share experiences, give each other feedback, and offer suggestions.
- *Instrumental groups:* Designed to assist members to maintain their level of function and meet health needs. Change, although it may occur, is not expected. The role of the leader is to select activities that meet the goals just described.

Educational groups deserve special mention owing to their popularity in both psychiatric and physical dysfunction settings. They typically fit in Mosey's (1981) "thematic group" category. These groups use a psychoeducational model and employ teaching approaches (Goldstein, Gershaw, and Spraflin, 1979; Kramer, 1984; Lillie and Armstrong, 1982). As Mosey (1981) explains, "These [thematic groups] may include performance components such as sensory integration or neuromuscular function or occupational performances such as activities of daily living or recreational/leisure skills" (p. 111). Ross' (1987, 1991; Ross and Burdick, 1981) "Structured Five-Stage Approach" is such a group approach aimed at physical/perceptual–motor, cognitive, and psychiatric conditions, as, for example, are groups structured with cognitive aims alone (Allen, 1985; Lundgren and Persechino, 1986).

The "directive group" (Kaplan, 1986, 1988), also a form of activity group, blends many of Mosey's (1981) types of activity groups. It is designed to help psychiatric patients who are functioning at a minimal level to adjust to group treatment regimens. Theoretically based on Kielhofner's Model of Human Occupation, the goals are aimed at "participation," "interaction," "attention," and "initiation" (Kaplan, 1988, pp. 48–49). Kaplan notes that the "directive group" is similar to Howe and Schwartzberg's 1986 functional group model, but the former is aimed at a more "basic level of competence." "For patients needing Directive Group, functional group approaches pick up where Directive Group leaves off" (Kaplan, 1988, p. 23).

Although the groups that Mosey describes as activity groups are usually considered occupational therapy groups, activity groups also include social work groups, such as those following the Vinter model (Galinsky and Schopler, 1974) and some groups in the field of nursing (Sampson and Marthas, 1981).

Theoretical perspective

The concept supporting the activity group has its roots in two different theoretical constructs: The first is the principle of group dynamics relating to how the curative factors in small groups bring about positive behavioral change; the second relates to the importance of "doing"—the role of purposeful activity in maintaining and developing skills.

Leader role

The role of the leader in the activity group would vary according to the particular group's goals (Box 1-18). The leader's responsibilities include (1) creating a group climate that facilitates interaction of group members, provides support for members, and relates group processes to the concerns of the members; (2) selecting appropriate activities or helping the group to do so; (3) structuring the activities for the group's level; (4) acting as a role model; and (5) guiding the learning of interpersonal and task skills. In most cases, the group is dependent on the leader to select and structure the task, particularly in the early stages of the group.

Box-18
Leader's Role

The leader's responsibilities typically include:

1. Creating a group climate
2. Selecting or helping select appropriate activities
3. Structuring activities for the group's level
4. Acting as a role model
5. Guiding skill learning

Group membership
In the selection of group members, a prospective member's cognitive, social, emotional, and perceptual–sensory skills need to be considered. In addition, one must consider the ability of the members to function in the spheres of work, play, and self-care. Depending on the goals of the particular group, a leader may select members who are similar or different in age, sex, sociocultural background, educational level, and identified problem areas.

Intrapsychic Groups

Group goals and structure
The general aim of intrapsychic groups is to achieve characterological and personality changes in each group member by "working through" the personal, intrapsychic, and historical antecedents of the present maladaptive personality patterns (Table 1-2). *Intrapsychic* refers to the processes and conflicts that occur within the individual. Insight into the unconscious and the self is the goal of psychoanalytic therapy. In addition to insight, groups can offer activity experiences that meet group needs and provide ego support for the members (Howe, 1968a, 1968b). Groups of this type include psychoanalytic therapy groups, projective occupational therapy groups, art therapy groups, and psychodrama groups.

Theoretical perspective
Intrapsychic groups are based primarily on psychoanalytic theory. The principles of psychoanalytic therapy are applied to the group setting, with the focus of observation and analysis placed mainly on the individual member, not on the group. Transference is a phenomenon that has particular importance in the

Table 1-2
Overview of the Intrapsychic Group Treatment Model

Type of Group	Examples	Group Goal	Theoretical Perspective	Leader Role	Membership
Intrapsychic group	Psychoanalytic therapy, projective occupational therapy, art therapy, psycho-drama groups	To achieve personality change through: 1) Insight (Slavson, 1950) 2) Tension reduction 3) Trans-ference	Psychoanalytic theory and activity group therapy Slavson, (1950) and transference	1) To explore and interpret personal member conflicts 2) To analyze free association	Requirements: 1) Intact ego 2) Ability to think abstractly 3) Homogenous or balanced heterogenous group

intrapsychic group. In projective occupational therapy groups and art therapy groups, object relations theory, including human and nonhuman objects, is also useful. In activity group therapy as developed by Slavson (1950), members work out their intrapsychic, preconscious conflicts through activities, and therapeutic results are obtained more through the discharge of tension inherent in the conflict than through insight.

Leader role

In these groups, the leader primarily guides members in their exploration, interpretation, and "working through" of personal conflicts. The leader may help individual members by validating and clarifying their perceptions of reality. Leader techniques include encouraging free association and analysis of transference. To encourage member participation, the leader might make available projective media, such as clay, paints, paper, or music. The group members are dependent on the leader for the analysis and interpretation of their behavior.

Group membership

Members must have a clear ego identity and cognitive ability to use the group to develop insight; that is, they should be able to deal in the realm of the abstract. In these groups, membership is usually homogeneous in age, sex, and socioeconomic status. Groups are carefully structured for a balance of problem areas and characterological style.

Social Systems Groups

Group goals and structure

The general aim of these groups is to help participants learn about group processes and dynamics through participation in a collective task experience (Table 1-3). "Our attention is directed to how relationships within groups are formed and how these relationships stabilize; how decisions are made; how patterns of behavior emerge; and how parts fit together to form the whole family, team, or group" (Sampson and Marthas, 1981, p. 125). Groups of this type include T-groups, laboratory methods groups, and other educational group laboratories.

Theoretical perspective

The principles behind social systems groups are drawn from systems theory and are applied to the concepts of group process and group dynamics. Kurt Lewin (1951) is frequently identified as the founder of this theoretical perspective. He described the behavior of individuals in terms of a system of paths, barriers, forces, and goals. He coined the term *life space,* which refers to the environment experienced by the individual or the group. A group has a life space in that it operates in a milieu within it plans activities and conducts its business. Lewin focused on the here-and-now activity of the group and the interaction with its environment at the present time.

Table 1-3
Overview of the Systems Group Treatment Model

Type of Group	Examples	Group Goal	Theoretical Perspective	Leader Role	Membership
Systems group	T-groups, laboratory methods group, and other educational group laboratories	To focus on the how of group behavior in the present	Systems theory as applied to group dynamics; Lewin (1954) life space and inter-action theory of human behavior	1) To participate as an expert member 2) To establish appropriate group climate for process analysis	1) Varies from group to group 2) Shared goal and views within the group

Leader role

The role of the leader is to participate in the group as a member–expert and to establish an environment appropriate for process analysis. The leader tries to keep member attention focused on the "how" rather than the "why" or on here-and-now events rather than on intrapsychic issues in the group's exploration of its processes relative to the task that it seeks to accomplish. The members' dependence on the leader is situational and transient.

Group membership

Because social systems groups are educational and do not focus on individual member concerns, the membership varies. Despite changing membership, there may be a single focus, concern, or goal for the group so that members can maintain the group.

Growth Groups

Group goals and structure

Growth groups are aimed at increasing members' sensitivity to feelings or enhancing members' ability to help themselves through the power of the group (Table 1-4). The precise methods by which these goals are accomplished vary from group to group, but all are aimed at personal growth through didactic and action-oriented experiences. According to Shaffer and Galinsky (1974), "The Encounter format offers an intensive group experience that is designed to put the normally alienated individual into closer contact—or 'encounter'—with himself, with others, and with the world of nature and pure sensation" (p. 211). Groups included in this category are encounter groups, sensitivity training groups, and marathon groups. Self-help groups also belong in this category, but they differ in that they are frequently conducted as leaderless groups.

Table 1-4
Overview of the Growth Group Treatment Model

Type of Group	Examples	Group Goal	Theoretical Perspective	Leader Role	Membership
Growth group	Encounter, sensitivity training, marathon, and self-help groups*	1) To increase member sensitivity to self and others 2) To learn through action-oriented experiences	Existential and humanistic concepts, as in Schutz (1967); Rogers (1961); Perls, Hefferline, and Goodman, (1971); and Maslow (1962)	1) To facilitate group interaction 2) To model behavior 3) To be a good resource	A self-selected homogenous group desiring increased awareness, personal growth, and empower-ment

* Self-help groups are frequently conducted as leaderless groups.

Peer support has been isolated as a distinctive feature of the type of help (Schwartzberg, 1994) offered in this type of group. Further, as Borg and Bruce (1991) note,

> Education has a major role in groups providing support and knowledge to manage chronic diseases (e.g., arthritis and diabetes). During these support groups, patients learn about the disease process and medical management of symptoms, get advice regarding problems related to the chronic illness, and gain support from group members as they share experiences and attempt problem-solving. (p. 7)

The role of occupational therapist as consultant to support groups is receiving increased attention (McConchie, 1989), as is the difference between occupational therapy treatment and this form of peer group help (Sacenti, 1988; Schulz, 1993, 1994; Schwartzberg, 1994). Because of the unique role of leader as facilitator, consultant, and resource person, this group is best categorized as a growth group. It can more closely resemble the activity group model when the occupational therapist assumes greater authority than the members of the group. This happens in acute care and rehabilitation facilities versus community settings.

Theoretical perspective
Growth groups are based on the principles of humanistic and existential philosophy and psychology that seek to fulfill the potential inherent in each person. These principles are explained in the writing of such leaders as Carl Rogers

(1961), William Schutz (1967), Fritz Perls (Perls, Hefferline, and Goodman, 1971), and Abraham Maslow (1962).

Leader role

The role of the leader in growth groups is to facilitate interaction, learning, and experience among the group members. The leader often teaches through a modeling process, for example, by modeling openness, spontaneity, the expression of feelings, and mutual aid. The group members are dependent on the leader only as a teacher or contributor to the group. Frequently, the leader is seen only as the person who initially organized the group.

Group membership

Members are individuals who seek a growth experience and will therefore share a desire for growth. Most likely members will range in age from adolescence to older adulthood.

Natural Groups

Although not included in the overview of group treatment models, natural groups also offer therapeutic properties and are part of prevention and intervention programs (Fig. 1-2). Examples of natural groups are families, church groups, work groups, community living groups, and interactive educational or recreational groups. These groups are found mainly in the community and are interactive in nature. The memberships of natural groups are usually not determined by the leader and may include persons of all ages. The group structure is

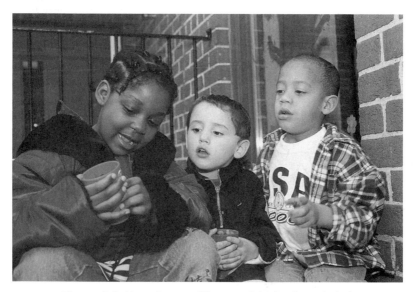

Figure 1-2. Natural group. (Photograph by Sarah Brezinsky.)

usually informal. The role of the leader is to facilitate interaction, support participation by members, and act as a teacher or contributor to the group to help it achieve its goals.

Conclusion

Various groups are available to meet the therapeutic and educational needs of individuals. The types of groups listed in this chapter do not exhaust the list of possibilities. Groups can be designed to suit any particular need or goal. Research has shown the types of interactions that group leaders can expect and has also indicated appropriate responses and techniques for dealing with these interactions.

Review Questions

1. What is meant by group cohesiveness? How may cohesiveness be identified in the group? How can a leader assist a group to be cohesive?
2. Should the group leader discuss his or her goals for the group with the members? After a discussion might the goals need to be altered, or even revised as the group continues to work together? If this happens, does this mean that the leader is ineffective?
3. Does the group composition limit the possibility of a group achieving specific goals? For instance, if the group goal is socialization, would the size of the group matter? Why? Would it matter if the group were open or closed? Voluntary or involuntary?
4. Seeing as how groups can be designed to serve any specific need or goal, why is it important to design a model specifically for occupational therapy groups?

References

Allen, C. K. (1985). Occupational Therapy for Psychiatric Diseases: Measurement and Management of Cognitive Disabilities. Boston: Little, Brown & Company.

Asch, S. E. (1960). Effects of group pressure upon the modification and distortion of judgments. In D. Cartwright and A. Zander (eds.), Group Dynamics: Research and Theory (2nd ed.). Evanston, IL: Row, Peterson, pp. 189–200.

Atkinson, J. W., and Feather, N. (1966). A Theory of Achievement Motivation. New York: John Wiley & Sons.

Back, K. (1951). Influence through social communication. Journal of Abnormal Psychology 46: 9–23.[3]

Bales, R. F. (1955a). Adaptive and integrative changes as sources of strain in social systems. In A. P. Hare, E. F. Borgatta, and R. F. Bales (eds.), Small Groups. New York: Knopf.

Bales, R. F. (1955b). The equilibrium problem in small groups. In A. P. Hare, E. F. Borgatta, and R. F. Bales (eds.), Small Groups, New York: Knopf.

Bales, R. F., and Borgatta, E. F. (1962). Size of group as a factor in the interaction profile. In A. P. Hare, E. F. Borgatta, and R. F. Bales (eds.), Small Groups (2nd ed.). New York: Knopf.

Bem, D., Wallach, M., and Kogan, N. (1965). Group decision making under risk of aversive consequences. Journal of Personal and Social Psychology 1: 453–460.

Benjamin, A. (1978). Behavior in Small Groups. Boston: Houghton Mifflin.

Benne, K., and Sheats, P. (1978). Functional roles of groups members. In L. Bradford (ed.), Group Development (2nd ed.). La Jolla, CA: University Associates, pp. 52–61.

Bennis, W. B., and Shepard, H. S. (1956). A theory of group development. Human Relations 9: 415–457.

Bion, W. R. (1959). Experiences in Groups. New York: Basic Books.

Borg, B., and Bruce, M. A. (1991). The Group System: The Therapeutic Activity Group in Occupational Therapy. Thorofare, NJ: Slack.

Bronfenbrenner, U. (1979). The Ecology of Human Development: Experiments by Nature and Design. Cambridge: Harvard University Press.

Buckley, W. (ed.). (1968). Modern Systems Research for the Behavioral Scientist. Chicago: Aldine.

Cartwright, D., and Zander, A. (1960). Group Dynamics: Research and Theory (2nd ed.). New York: Harper & Row, pp. 69–92.

Castore, G. F. (1962). Number of verbal interrelationships as a determinant of group size. Journal of Abnormal Social Psychology 64: 456–457.

Cooley, C. H. (1909). Social Organization: A Study of the Larger Mind. New York: Scribner's.

Corey, G., and Corey, M. S. (1977). Groups: Process and Practice (2nd ed.). Monterey, CA: Brooks/Cole.

Corsini, R., and Rosenberg, B. (1955). Mechanisms of group psychotherapy: Process and dynamics. Journal of Abnormal and Social Psychology 15: 406–411.

Deutsch, M. (1960). The effects of cooperation and competition upon group process. In D. Cartwright and A. Zander (eds.), Group Dynamics: Research and Theory (2nd ed.). New York: Harper & Row, pp. 461–482.

Dion, K. L., Miller, N., and Magnan, M. (1970). Cohesiveness and social responsibility as determinants of group risk taking. Proceedings of the Annual Convention of the American Psychological Association 5(Part I): 335–336.

Donigian, J., and Malnati, R. (1997). Systemic Group Therapy: A Triadic Model. Pacific Grove, CA: Brooks/Cole.

Falk-Kessler, J., Momich, C., and Perel, S. (1991). Therapeutic factors in occupational therapy groups. American Journal of Occupational Therapy 45(1): 59–66.

Festinger, L., and Thibaut, J. (1951). Interpersonal communication in small groups. Journal of Abnormal and Social Psychology 16: 92–99.

Fidler, G. (1969). The task-oriented group as a context for treatment. American Journal of Occupational Therapy 23: 43–48.

Finn, M. (1989). Patients' perceptions of occupational therapy groups: Interview generated factors. Unpublished master's thesis, Tufts University–Boston School of Occupational Therapy, Medford, MA.

Frank, J. D. (1957). Some determinants, manifestations, and effects of cohesiveness in therapy groups. International Journal of Group Psychotherapy 7: 53–63.

Galinsky, M. J., and Schopler, J. H. (1974). The social work group. In J. B. Shaffer and M. D. Galinsky (eds.), Models of Group Therapy and Sensitivity Training. Englewood Cliffs, NJ: Prentice-Hall, pp. 19–48.

Garland, J. A., Jones, H. E., and Kolodny, R. (1965). A model for stages of development in social work groups. In S. Bernstein (ed.), Explorations in Group Work. Boston: Boston University School of Social Work.

Goldstein, A. P., Gershaw, N. J., and Spraflin, R. P. (1979). Structured learning therapy: Development and evaluation. American Journal of Occupational Therapy 33(10): 635–639.

Hare, A. P. (1962). Handbook of Small Group Research. New York: Free Press of Glencoe.

Horwitz, M. (1960). The recall of interrupted group tasks: An experimental study of individual motivation in relation to group goals. In D. Cartwright and A. Zander (eds.), Group Dynamics: Research and Theory (2nd ed.). New York: Harper & Row, pp. 444–460.

Howe, M. (1968a). An occupational therapy activity group. American Journal of Occupational Therapy 22: 176–179.

Howe, M. (1968b). A review of selected professional literature describing four youth groups to determine structure with reference to psychiatric occupational therapy. Unpublished master's thesis, San Jose State University, San Jose, CA.

Hurwitz, J. I., Zander, A., and Hymovitch, B. (1960). Some effects of power on the relations among group members. In D. Cartwright and A. Zander (eds.), Group Dynamics: Research and Theory (2nd ed.). New York: Harper & Row, pp. 291–297.

Kaplan, K. (1986). The directive group: Short-term treatment for psychiatric patients with a minimal level of functioning. American Journal of Occupational Therapy 40(7): 474–481.

Kaplan, K. L. (1988). Directive Group Therapy Innovative Mental Health Treatment. Thorofare, NJ: Slack.

Knowles, M., and Knowles, H. (1959). Introduction to Group Dynamics. New York: Association Press.

Kramer, L. W. (1984). SCORE: Solving community obstacles and restoring employment. Occupational Therapy in Mental Health: A Journal of Psychosocial Practice and Research 4(1): 1–135.

Lewin, K. (1951). Field Theory in Social Science. New York: Harper & Row.

Lewin, K., Lippitt, R., and White, R. (1939). Patterns of aggressive behavior in experimentally created social climates. Journal of Social Psychology 10: 271–299.

Lifton, W. M. (1961). Working with Groups: Group Process and Individual Growth. New York: John Wiley & Sons.

Lillie, M., and Armstrong, H. (1982). Contributions to the development of psychoeducational approaches to mental health service. American Journal of Occupational Therapy 36(7): 438–443.

Lippitt, G. L. (1961). How to get results from a group. In L. P. Bradford (ed.), Group Development. Washington, DC: National Training Laboratories, National Education Association.

Loeser, L. H. (1957). Some aspects of group dynamics. International Journal of Group Psychotherapy 7 (1): 5–19.

Lundgren, C. C., and Persechino, E. L. (1986). Cognitive group: A treatment program for head injured adults. American Journal of Occupational Therapy 40(6): 397–401.

Maslow, A. (1962). Toward a Psychology of Being. Princeton, NJ: Van Nostrand.

McConchie, S. D. (December 1989) Establishing support and advocacy groups. Mental Health Special Interest Section Newsletter, pp. 5–6, 8. Rockville, MD: American Occupational Therapy Association.

Mosey, A. C. (1973). Activities Therapy. New York: Raven Press.

Mosey, A. C. (1981). Occupational Therapy: Configuration of a Profession. New York: Raven Press.

Napier, R., and Gershenfeld, M. K. (1973). Groups: Theory and Experience. Boston: Houghton Mifflin.

Nelson, D. L. (1997). Why the profession of occupational therapy will flourish in the 21st century. American Journal of Occupational Therapy 51(1): 12.

Perls, F., Hefferline, R. E., and Goodman, P. (1971). Gestalt Therapy. New York: Bantam.

Raven, B. H., and Rietsema, J. (1957). The effects of varied clarity of group goal and group path upon the individual and his relation to his group. Human Relations 10: 29–44.

Rogers, C. (1961). On Becoming a Person. Boston: Houghton Mifflin.

Ross, M. (1987). Group Process Using Therapeutic Activities in Chronic Care. Thorofare, NJ: Slack.

Ross, M. (1991). Integrative Group Therapy: The Structured Five-Stage Approach (2nd ed.). Thorofare, NJ: Slack.

Ross, M., and Burdick, D. (1981). Sensory Integration: A Training Manual for Therapists and Teachers for Regressed, Psychiatric and Geriatric Patient Groups. Thorofare, NJ: Slack.

Sacenti, L. (1988). Mastery and levels of participation in members of two groups for chronic pain: Self-help and professionally led. Unpublished master's thesis, Tufts University–Boston School of Occupational Therapy, Medford, MA.

Sampson, E., and Marthas, M. (1981). Group Process for the Health Professions (2nd ed.). New York: John Wiley & Sons.

Schulz, C. (1993). A member perspective on a support group for head injury. Unpublished master's thesis, Tufts University–Boston School of Occupational Therapy, Medford, MA.

Schulz, C. H. (1994). Helping factors in a peer-developed support group for persons with head injury, part 2: Survivor interview perspective. American Journal of Occupational Therapy 48(4): 305–309.

Schutz, W. C. (1960). FIRO: A Three-Dimensional Theory of Interpersonal Behavior. New York: Rinehart, Winston.

Schutz, W. C. (1967). Joy: Expanding Human Awareness. New York: Grove Press.

Schwartzberg, S. L. (1994). Helping factors in a peer-developed support group for persons with head injury, part 1: Participant observer perspective. American Journal of Occupational Therapy 48(4): 297–304.

Shaefer, C., Johnson, L., and Wherry, J. (1982). Group Therapies for Children and Youth. San Francisco: Jossey-Bass.

Shaffer, J. B., and Galinsky, M. D. (1974). Models of Group Therapy and Sensitivity Training. Englewood Cliffs, NJ: Prentice-Hall.

Slavson, S. R. (1950). Analytic Group Psychotherapy with Children, Adolescents, and Adults. New York: Columbia University Press.

Tubbs, S. (1984). A Systems Approach to Small Group Interaction. New York: Random House.

Tuckman, B. W. (1965). Developmental sequence in small groups. Psychological Bulletin 63: 384–399.

Von Bertalanffy, L. (1968). General Systems Theory: Foundations, Development, Application (rev. ed). New York: George Braziller.

Webster, D. (1988). Patients' perceptions of therapeutic factors in occupational therapy groups. Unpublished master's thesis, Tufts University–Boston School of Occupational Therapy, Medford, MA.

Webster, D., and Schwartzberg, S. L. (1992). Patients' perception of curative factors in occupational therapy groups. Occupational Therapy in Mental Health: A Journal of Psychosocial Practice and Research 12(1): 3–24.

Yalom, I. D. (1970). The Theory and Practice of Group Psychotherapy. New York: Basic Books.

Yalom, I. D. (1975). The Theory and Practice of Group Psychotherapy (2nd ed.). New York: Basic Books.

Yalom, I. D. (1983). Inpatient Group Psychotherapy. New York: Basic Books.

Zander, A., and Havelin, A. (1960). Social comparison and intergroup attraction. Human Relations 13: 21–32.

Chapter 2
History of Occupational Therapy Group Treatment

- Project Era: 1922–1936
- Socialization Era: 1937–1953
- Group Dynamics–Process Era: 1954–1961
- Ego Building–Psychodynamic Era: 1962–1969
- Adaptation Era: 1970s–1990s
- Conclusion
- Review Questions
- References

Occupational therapists have been using groups in their treatment plans since the 1920s, and today the group can be found as a treatment tool in all areas of occupational therapy. As the use of group treatment increased in all specialties of occupational therapy during the 20th century, the role of the occupational therapist and the nature of the group as a treatment tool changed. In Chapter 1 we examined several different types of groups. The state of current practice will be addressed in Chapter 3, and in Chapter 4 we shall present a model of the functional approach to group work. In this chapter we shall examine the history of group work in occupational therapy, investigating the trends and forces leading to the occupational therapy group as it is known today.

The history of group work in occupational therapy falls into five periods or eras: (1) the project era, (2) the socialization era, (3) the group dynamics–process era, (4) the ego building–psychodynamic era, and (5) the adaptation era. As we explore the development of groups as a treatment tool, we should keep in mind the following questions:

1. How did occupational therapy evolve over time?
2. What forces led to the shift in occupational therapy from an individualized to a collective approach?
3. How did group treatment contribute to the development of occupational therapy?
4. How does group treatment fit into the occupational therapy profession as a whole?

Although the history of group work as an acknowledged tool of occupational therapists does not officially begin until 1922, when Adolph Meyer (1922/1977) described the use of individual craft projects in a group setting, using group work as a tool for healing already had a long if unappreciated history in Western civilization (Box 2-1). Occupational therapy was practiced long before it was given its "20th century name," to use Bockoven's (1971) expression. Kielhofner and Burke (1977) also noted that "the use of occupation as a form of treatment for the physically or mentally ill is documented throughout recorded history" (p. 678).

The moral treatment movement of the 19th century is cited most often as the immediate historical origin of occupational therapy (Bing, 1981; Bockoven, 1971; Gillette and Kielhofner, 1979; Kielhofner and Burke, 1977). The moral treatment movement emerged from the humanitarian trends of the 18th and 19th centuries (Gillette and Kielhofner, 1979; Kielhofner and Burke, 1977). The objective of this movement was to correct attitudes and habits of living. "The physical, temporal, and social environment was engineered so as to correct faculty [sic] habits of living and regenerate new ones. . . . It employed the moral remedies of education, daily habits, work, and play as therapeutic processes for normalizing disorganized behavior in the mentally ill" (Kielhofner and Burke, 1977, p. 678). The patients' programs apparently included individual and collective activities. The group activities were orchestrated solely by the therapist. In describing an aspect of his program in Paris in 1840, Leuret presented group activity as it might have appeared to the casual observer:

> To some I assign reading out loud, reading verses or singing. Reading is usually performed by several patients who recite alternate passages or sentences from a story according to a plan which I have devised. . . . Some do not enter into this exercise with much cooperation, but pray or grumble instead. (1840/1948, p. 64)

As he continues his description, he discusses goals and achievements that are still sought by therapists today:

> Once they overcome their initial distaste, stimulated by the example of others and by the presence of an audience, they begin to apply themselves to the work which they eventually accept with pleasure. Those who read well, drill others and soon their self-esteem improves and they become better teachers than I could ever be. (Leuret, 1840/1948, p. 64)

The goals and procedures Leuret used are remarkably similar to those used by occupational therapists today. He apparently structured the activity and group

---

Box 2-1
Before His Time

Licht (1948) pointed out that Asclepiades, who was born more than 100 years before Christ, was the first physician to recommend activity as a treatment for patients with mental illness. He advised physicians to treat patients "safely, quickly, pleasantly" (p. 1).

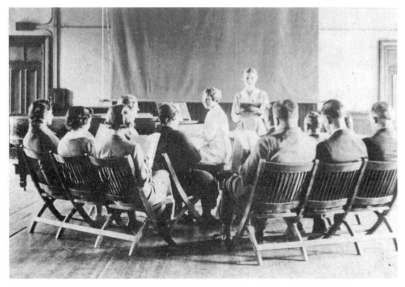

Figure 2-1. A singing group. (Courtesy of the Boston School of Occupational Therapy Archives, Tufts University, Medford, MA.)

processes according to what is now called a developmental continuum. The proponents of the 19th century moral treatment movement thus strongly influenced the practice of early 20th century pioneers in occupational therapy by serving as models (Fig. 2-1).

Project Era: 1922–1936

Identifying when and by whom the first occupational therapy groups were conducted is a difficult task. Perhaps the confusion stems from the numerous definitions of group treatment or from the failure of therapists to identify their practice as group treatment. Most likely, the first occupational therapy groups were groups of patients working on individual activities in a clinic or on a ward. They were probably an organized unit but not necessarily a group with a unified goal or interdependent tasks. This unit can be called a collective, whereas a unit with a unified goal or interdependent tasks is more strictly defined as a group (Box 2-2).

Box 2-2
Varied Settings

The collective offers a setting that is most similar to individual therapy, and the group provides a setting with a strong sense of group centeredness.

This nature of the collective unit, as opposed to the group, dominated the years between 1922 and 1936, giving rise to the name of this period. During these early years, the members in a collective focused on individual projects, which were completed in the open setting of the collective (Fig. 2-2). There was little or no emphasis on the process of interaction taking place among the mem-

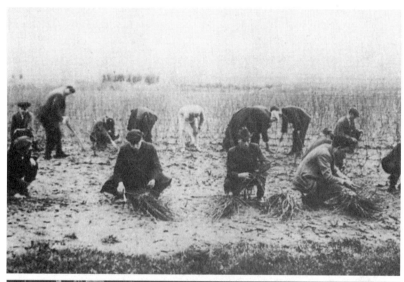

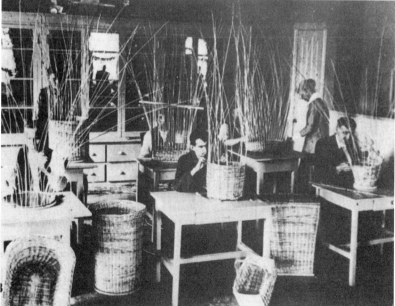

Figure 2-2. Occupational therapy collectives. (Courtesy of the Boston School of Occupational Therapy Archives, Tufts University, Medford, MA.)

bers of the collective while they worked on their individual projects in the company of others.

During the early years of the 20th century, there was enough interest in this sort of activity to lead therapists to found a professional organization. In 1917, the National Society for the Promotion of Occupational Therapy was founded (Reed and Sanderson, 1980). Five years later, in 1922, the first official journal of occupational therapy was published. In the first issue of the *Archives of Occupational Therapy,* Adolph Meyer (1922/1977) and Eleanor Clarke Slagle (1922) individually described occupational therapy collectives. Meyer (1922/1977) observed the following:

> It had long been interesting to see how groups of a few excited patients can be seated in a corner in a small circle of two or three settees and kept wonderfully contented picking the hair of mattresses, or doing simple tasks not too readily arousing the desire for big movements and uncontrollable excitement and yet not too taxing to their patience. Groups of patients with raffia and basket work, or with various kinds of handwork and weaving and bookbinding and metal and leather work, took the place of the bored wall flowers and of mischiefmakers. (p. 640)

Similarly, Slagle (1922) suggested a program that included collectives. Slagle advised moving the patient through a series of four steps. The steps progressed from individual habit training, to the "kindergarten group" for "stimulating the special senses," to occupational therapy ward classes focusing on the individual, and finally, to the "occupational center," or "curative workshop," for helping the patient adapt to other members of the group (pp. 15–16). In the final phase, the patient was moved from supervised activity to a collective focusing on vocational goals. Slagle called this the "preindustrial group" (p. 16).

Both Meyer and Slagle viewed the activities in collectives as a means for patients to develop socially acceptable habits to replace their pathological reactions. Thus, the Project Era begins with a formalization of the philosophy of 19th century moral treatment. This formalization, however, was only one thread from the previous century influencing 20th century professionals.

During the last decades of the 19th century, historically named the Progressive Era, America was becoming a scientific and industrialized society (Wiebe, 1967). There were an increase in scientific concerns, developments in technology, booming industrialism, increased urbanization and immigration, and a shift from shop to factory in industry (Wiebe, 1967). Women were fighting for the right to work in an occupation of their choice (Smuts, 1959). According to Wiebe (1967), these changes called for a new set of values and a new kind of social order.

Like many other institutions, hospitals changed during this period, and these changes had a crucial impact on the developing health professions. Rosner (1979) points out that because of the economic and social forces of the depression of the 1890s, hospitals changed from charity institutions to paying institutions: "The move away from charity to pay services was rationalized as part of the larger Progressive Era movements toward order, efficiency and bureaucracy" (pp. 118–119). By 1922, when Meyer and Slagle described occupational therapy, these forces had already had an effect. Patients now did part of the labor of the institution (Box 2-3).

As early as 1923, a therapist surmised that there was an economic rationale for prescribing work as occupational therapy. Canton (1923) stated:

> It is interesting to note that work originally was given only to state patients, planned to relieve employees rather than to effect cures, and managed from the viewpoint of utility. It was found that other patients wished to share in these employments and since the relatives who were paying for their care sanctioned the arrangement, they too, were permitted to putter around so that now the proper use of time in some helpful and gratifying activity has become a fundamental issue in the treatment of all neuro-psychiatric patients. (p. 348)

The recognition of a connection between activity and health could have led to several results, not only to the collectives in which members worked on projects but also on minor jobs for the institution in which they lived. The path through this development, however, is reasonably clear and direct. If we examine the founders and early practitioners in this field, we can perhaps understand the choice of emphasizing collective or group work over jobs or products.

When the National Society for the Promotion of Occupational Therapy was formed in 1917, its membership included medical doctors, social workers, teachers, nurses, and artists (Hopkins, 1978). Most of the members were women, and this was in character with the times. "The proportion of all women workers who were professionals grew from 11.9 per cent in 1920 to 14.2 per cent in 1930" (Chafe, 1972, pp. 89–90). The role of women in founding and defining occupational therapy is sometimes neglected in historical analyses, leading to the false conclusion that occupational therapy is similar to the male-dominated professions in healthcare. In fact, women in occupational therapy shaped the direction the field took in this early era, choosing collective work because of their backgrounds (Box 2-4).

There was no mention of groups in the occupational therapy literature from 1923 to 1936, but in 1936, 14 years after Meyer's and Slagle's papers were first published, an interest in groups reappeared. Three papers on occupational therapy group treatment were published in 1936. These articles present evidence that therapists were beginning to conceive of the gathering of pa-

---

Box 2-3
Cheap Labor

According to Rothman (1980), activities necessary for the daily operation of the hospital, such as farming, laundry, and sewing, were called occupational therapy. The occupational therapy collective thus became an economic unit in which the patient was also a worker.

Box 2-4
Founding Women

Occupational therapy began as a female-dominated profession. These founding women were likely to be from upper-class families and to be familiar with handicrafts and family or group living. They were also probably quite comfortable directing groups of people in a collective milieu.

tients as a group rather than only as a collective. Further, therapists were now dividing responsibility for a single project among several patients and viewing opportunities for involvement in a project as a device for restoring health.

Although the role of occupational therapy was not specified, L. Cody Marsh (1936) advocated that relatives of psychotic patients be given group treatment. Davis and Dunton, in 1936, as mentioned by Gleave (1947), described a form of mass occupational therapy in which patients had the opportunity to associate with a group project and to increase their self-respect through the group's accomplishment. To improve the use of group activity, Anderson (1936) suggested "project work," or "individualized group therapy." In project work, the therapist structures an activity to meet the group member's individual needs while still requiring each member to contribute to a larger group project.

Anderson (1936) emphasized that project work should not be confused with the activity usually offered by occupational therapy departments:

> Project work, with its designated therapeutic aims and offered for its therapeutic values, must not be confused with that type of group activity often provided in many institutions as a part of "hospital economy," "doing odd jobs," time filling activity, or furnishing labor needs of the institution with no reference to the value of the work for the individual concerned. Nor is project work the same as occupational therapy where the guest usually works in a group or alone on an individual project but not with the responsibility of contributing a part to a project which is the divided responsibility of an entire group. (p. 265)

This is the first clear indication that group work should be defined according to the patient and not according to the hospital and its economic needs or according to the physician's or therapist's interests.

Anderson (1936) clearly departed from the norm when he suggested occupational therapy should focus on the patients' therapeutic needs rather than fulfilling the institution's labor needs. Nevertheless, he emphasized that the therapist was responsible for carrying out the physicians' "therapeutic aims" and should regularly report to them. These "therapeutic aims," using Anderson's terms, were to "provide an outlet for aggressions," "permit propitiation of guilt," "provide freedom for fantasy expression," and "permit opportunity to create" (p. 265).

> **Box 2-5**
> **Building Credibility**
>
> Between 1922 and 1936, the focus was on the development of occupational therapy as a profession.

The reports and advances by Anderson and others came after more than 10 years of silence. Why did it take so long for group treatment to be mentioned again in the occupational therapy literature? Why was the process of development a slow one? The following writers may give us some answers to these questions.

In her historical analysis of the development of occupational therapy, Woodside (1971) pointed out that between 1910 and 1929, occupational therapy developed into an active and organized profession. The first set of minimal educational standards were published in 1923; occupational therapy schools became affiliated with colleges and universities in the 1920s; and occupational therapists were first required to be registered with a specific set of credentials in 1929. According to Rerek (1971), the profession defined its direction in the mid-1930s by asking the American Medical Association to establish standards for occupational therapy education and to accredit each new school (Box 2-5). This, Rerek assumed, was when the profession formally assumed a medical ancillary role.

The climate of the mid-1930s stimulated professionals to reconsider the form of occupational therapy group treatment. During the depression, many occupational therapy departments closed, decreased their personnel, or struggled with limited supplies (Reed and Sanderson, 1980; Rerek, 1971). By this time, the field of medicine had become more "professionalized" and had increased its interest in scientific pursuits (Markowitz and Rosner, 1979). In addition, the harsh realities of the depression meant fewer women could enter male-dominated careers (Chafe, 1972). The limited number of jobs that did exist were given to men as they were the primary wage earners in households. More and more women turned to those areas of the economy that were traditionally open to them. This led to an increase in the number of aspiring professional women in services related to other professions (Box 2-6).

> **Box 2-6**
> **Growing Legacy**
>
> Women, with training in handicrafts and group techniques, filled the ranks of the occupational therapy profession and continued to shape the field throughout the 1930s.

It should not be surprising, then, that Rothman (1980) found in the 1930s that "the most popular and prevalent form of hospital 'treatment' throughout these years remained occupational therapy" (p. 344). According to Rothman (1980), "for most inmates, occupational therapy involved daily assignments to endless chores, chores as meaningless to their lives as they were important to the survival of the institution" (p. 346). Patients were not yet free from an economic role. Jobs were selected because they were necessary for the maintenance of the institution, not because of any specific interests or treatment goals for the patients. Rothman (1980) emphasized that "occupational therapy . . . was more than an occasional patient weaving or joining the wheelbarrow brigade. As in correctional institutions, it affected the very existence of the mental hospital, for inmate labor was essential to day-to-day maintenance of the facility" (p. 346).

Occupational therapy group treatment was clearly a development of the times. Hospitals established to treat patients also needed patient labor. The strong interest of women in the profession shaped the content and structure of that labor. Because women were taught many crafts as part of their upbringing, they were perhaps most able to teach inexpensive craft activities to groups of dependents, as well as to supervise group tasks of maintenance. Canton (1923) noted earlier in occupational therapy the aide must be both a teacher and a nurse:

> She will be the kind of person who needs the little touches which would make even the most barren place a bit homelike, and a certain amount of buzzing activity which is part of every normal environment. . . . In addition she must bring to the work the ability to teach certain projects now accepted as valuable occupations." (p. 355)

Finally, the willingness of female therapists to conduct group treatment under male supervision gave the physician, who was usually male, more time to pursue his new scientific and professional interests. As these elements combined to shape the outer form of the profession, researchers in the field were laying the groundwork for changes in the internal form of treatment.

Anderson (1936) was probably the first to identify a therapy group structure that would change behavior. In his view, the group is seen as a curative tool rather than as a way to keep patients occupied. In Anderson's project group, the elements of activity and group process foster personality change (Fig. 2-3). Anderson (1936) stated that group activities can fulfill ordinary health needs as well as therapeutic aims:

> In project work the guest actively participates as a member of a group in work, provided as far as practicable out of doors, which is of value to the entire group. Therapeutic aims, which may be to provide an outlet for aggressions, permit propitiation of guilt, provide freedom for fantasy expression, permit opportunity to create, and others designated by the psychiatrist in charge of the guest are followed for each individual and this permits and makes necessary individualization of the work within the larger group. In addition to the therapeutic values determined upon a psychiatric basis, this out-of-door activ-

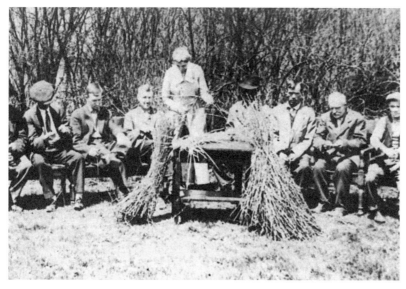

Figure 2-3. A project group. (Courtesy of the Boston School of Occupational Therapy Archives, Tufts University, Medford, MA.)

ity has the additional advantage of being physical exercise performed in the open air and sunshine. (p. 265)

Anderson's new vision of group therapy brought to an end the formative era that had called attention to the economic, as well as to the therapeutic, value of treating patients in groups (Box 2-7).

Socialization Era: 1937–1953

From 1937 to 1953, the literature on occupational therapy continued to grow (Box 2-8). Occupational therapy groups afforded patients an outlet for social needs and a vehicle for experiencing gratification from positive social contact. This period of group history is therefore called the Socialization Era.

In 1937, Dunton described quilt making as a group activity that aided socialization. Blackman (1940) later supported using a literary club for group treatment of schizophrenics (Fig. 2-4). The club's purpose was to work out "so-

> **Box 2-7**
> **Coming of Age**
>
> By the end of the Project Era, the occupational therapy group was a recognized tool for achieving prescribed therapeutic aims.

> ### Box 2-8
> ### Groups Evolved
>
> During the period from 1936-1953, the purpose of groups changed from individual activities to an environment providing opportunities for socialization among psychiatric patients.

cial cravings." In 1947 two publications described groups for socialization purposes. Lockerbie and Stevenson (1947) noted that group activities and clubs are valuable for socialization problems found in psychiatric hospitals. Basing her work on Slavson's group therapy approach, G. Margaret Gleave (1947), an occupational therapist, suggested using group therapy with children to provide a permissive, socializing atmosphere.

Slavson has been called the father of group psychotherapy (Schiffer, 1979); he also had a major influence on group treatment in occupational therapy, and his ideas were especially influential during this period. In 1934 Slavson designed his first group treatment method for children (Schiffer, 1979) based on the group work he conducted from 1911 to 1930. According to Schiffer (1979), "these [Slavson's] earlier groups were concerned primarily with the personal

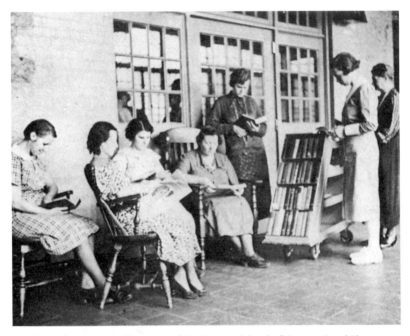

Figure 2-4. A literary club. (Courtesy of the Boston School of Occupational Therapy Archives, Tufts University, Medford, MA.)

> Box 2-9
> **Following Suit**
>
> It is likely that occupational therapists followed the lead of Slavson, the so-called "father of group psychotherapy," in their use of activity groups for socialization purposes during the 1940s.

enrichment of individuals through active participation in creative pursuits" (p. xiii). In about 1934, Slavson drew important conclusions about the curative effects of creative activities in a peer group environment (Box 2-9). Schiffer (1979) reported what Slavson told him in an interview at the time:

> He finally confirmed his original premise: it was the element of *compresence*, the actuality of being and interacting one with the other in the peer group, the sense of self-worth gained from newly acquired skills, the self-selected, completed craft and art projects, fortified by the spontaneous praise of fellow members, and the improved social status that were responsible for the corrective effects on personality and character. (pp. xvi–xvii)

Let us now examine the work of therapists during this period. Hyde, York, and Wood (1948) viewed games as an effective means for improving the socialization of psychiatric patients in a mental hospital (Fig. 2-5). White (1953) dis-

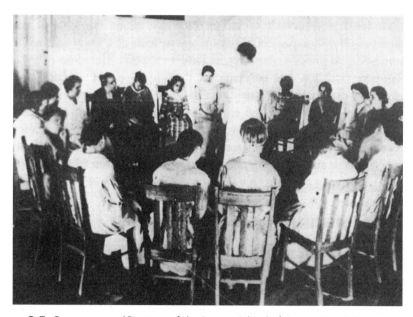

Figure 2-5. Group games. (Courtesy of the Boston School of Occupational Therapy Archives, Tufts University, Medford, MA.)

cussed the use of simplified repetitive activities that can include large groups of patients and can be structured for maximum involvement. Koven and Shuff (1953) found that guided group activity, such as gardening, painting, and museum trips, promotes cooperation, social awareness, and a sense of gratification through group achievement.

Taking a somewhat different approach, Halle and Landy (1948) recommended the integration of group activities used in occupational therapy such as craft and art activities with group psychotherapy. They found that the subject matter in the art activities group often correlated with the subjects being discussed by the psychiatrist in group psychotherapy. In 1947, Solomon and Fentress described "dramatized psychodynamics" in analytically oriented group psychotherapy. The authors discussed the technique of dramatization of psychodynamics but not its use in, or relationship to, occupational therapy groups.

These group techniques were developed and implemented during the Depression of the 1930s and during World War II and its aftermath (Rerek, 1971; Jantzen, 1972) (Box 2-10). The severe budget cuts of the 1930s were followed by an increased demand for therapists during World War II (Box 2-11). During World War II, 13 occupational therapy education programs were founded in association with established colleges or universities (Jantzen, 1972). Before World War II, there were only five educational programs; three were in independent proprietary schools, one was in a hospital, and only one was in an undergraduate liberal arts college (Jantzen, 1972). The 1940s brought new programs in this field to the forefront of educational growth.

The 1940s saw tremendous growth in occupational therapy programs despite budget cuts. Groups enabled therapists to treat a greater number of patients within a limited time. Because there was still relatively little theoretical orientation, occupational therapists remained in need of supervision and continued to serve an ancillary role. As an extension of the physician, the therapist could treat many patients at a lower cost while continuing to provide necessary medical treatment. The close relation between medicine and occupational therapy no doubt explains why physicians dominated the articles in this field. Of nine occupational therapy journal papers published on occupational therapy group treatment during this period, four were published by male physicians, three were coauthored by a male physician and a female occupational therapist, and only two were authored by female occupational therapists.

Group Dynamics–Process Era: 1954–1961

The 1950s brought a shift in occupational therapy group treatment. Professionals now recognized the group's curative powers and sought to use these powers to achieve therapeutic goals. Therapists or leaders were also structuring their role and the group's membership and activities to meet various patients' needs (Box 2-12).

These changes resulted in part from two factors. First, occupational therapists were now exposed in their training to the concept of group dynamics. Therapists learned how to manipulate a group to achieve specific therapeutic aims. They learned that the group could be used as an environment to produce change in, or support for, specific kinds of behavior. This was indeed an era of group dynamics and process. Second, the introduction of somatic therapies, particularly drugs, enabled patients to function more easily in social settings, thereby freeing the therapist of the earlier concern for socialization and maintenance (Feuss and Maltby, 1959). Therapists could now concentrate on treating specific problems of individual patients and developing new forms of the group to meet those needs.

In 1954, Fidler and Fidler proposed ways that groups could facilitate treatment; they suggested a new concept of occupational therapy as a laboratory for experimentation of behavior. This concept and its model differed from previous models because Fidler and Fidler recognized the curative effects of the learning, practicing, and modeling of healthy interpersonal behaviors that occurred naturally in an occupational therapy group. Recognizing the limitations of verbal groups for helping chronic psychotic patients, Bobis, Harrison, and Traub (1955) observed the progress of patients in an occupational therapy activity group: "Group projects were emphasized with patients working together

---

Box 2-12
Process in Action

In the 1950s, therapists no longer assumed that all patients in group treatment had the same needs.

> **Box 2-13**
> **Specialized Groups**
>
> Activity group therapy seemed to be the more effective method for chronic, nonverbal psychotic patients.

or doing different parts of a project. Suggestion was used a great deal by the occupational therapist—steady, gentle urging to participate in the group or group project" (p. 20). Patients showed a higher adjustment level in the activity group setting; the authors concluded that the group played an important role in the patients' improvement (Box 2-13).

Nelson and colleagues (1956) developed groups for differing types of patients, diagnoses, goals, and objectives. They structured "group occupational therapy" for, among others, insulin patients, postlobotomy patients, and male geriatric patients. A graded group program was designed especially for women. Patients were selected for one of three groups according to their level of adjustment. The group members were homogeneous in their level of ability rather than in their diagnoses, which enabled them to benefit from socialization opportunities in a particular group structure (Box 2-14). Combs (1959) designed activities for a custodial care group of elderly men in a chronic disease hospital, structuring them so that the patients moved from activities primarily concerned with individual performance to ones concerned with group performance.

In 1958, an experimental sheltered workshop program was implemented in a home for the aged. Because the authors believed that "for the group as a whole, work for which one is paid is worthwhile activity" (Lakin and Dray, 1958, p. 173), wage earning activity was structured into a group situation as a therapeutic modality. There were several positive effects for the group, including maintenance of adequate self-image and increased social contact.

Springfield and Tullis (1958) conducted a pilot study to determine a method for resocializing chronic patients. The average period of continuous hospitalization for these patients was 31 years, and all subjects were charac-

> **Box 2-14**
> **Grading by Ability**
>
> The occupational therapist's role ranged from a passive participant in the higher level group to the active encourager who meets needs and structures activity in the lower group.

teristically apathetic. The researchers found improvement was more noticeable in the activity group than during times when the project was not being conducted. Springfield and Tullis (1958) noted, "We were fully aware that if our program was to succeed, the emphasis must be placed on interpersonal relations rather than on any special activity" (p. 248).

Moss and Stewart (1959) developed a program for geriatric patients to facilitate movement from hospital to community. They developed groups for particular patient needs. "The patients were divided into treatment groups according to their specific disabilities or needs" (Moss and Stewart, 1959, p. 268). For example, one group of patients with organic disorders was given training in self-care activities, whereas a group of confused and withdrawn patients was given simple individual tasks that they could successfully complete because they needed motivation and reassurance. After several months in generalized activities, the therapist suggested that the patients work on one group project. In a similar project, the therapist chose eight men who could benefit from intensive group activity. The group worked on one large project rather than on smaller individual projects related to a common goal.

The 1950s were also a period of increased theoretical research and publishing. The American Occupational Therapy Association conducted an institute on the theme of "interpersonal relationships" (AOTA, 1955) (Box 2-15). Similarly, Gibb (1958) wrote on general group process principles for occupational therapists. He described how to make groups more effective using concepts of group dynamics as guiding principles. The 1956 Allenberry Workshop held a conference on the function and preparation of the psychiatric occupational therapist, and Wilma West (1959) edited the proceedings. Participants made recommendations for the education of the occupational therapist in the use of group techniques, the psychodynamics of interpersonal relationships in a group, group dynamics, use of the therapist as a therapeutic tool, and selection of group activities. There was discussion of the function of the psychiatric occupational therapist. It should not be surprising that in the 1950s "the majority of [occupational therapy] schools felt that teaching group relations is of

---

Box 2-15
Defining Theory

The theme of the American Occupational Therapy Association's institute in 1955 was "interpersonal relationships." Topics such as "Diagnosing Factors in Interpersonal Relationships," "Developing Effective Patterns of Leadership," and "Understanding the Complexities of Staff Relationships" were discussed. Types of leadership, functions of leadership, group dynamics and factors, and group processes were included. The proceedings of the institute were published for the association membership in the American Journal of Occupational Therapy.

major and vital importance . . . that their students need both theory and practice in groups" (West, 1959, p. 173).

By the early 1960s, papers on group treatment were emphasizing the importance of the interpersonal relationship between the occupational therapist and patient and the role of activity in fostering patient adjustment (Fidler and Fidler, 1960; Gratke and Lux, 1960; Novick, 1961). This practice also received empirical support. In 1959, Efron, Marks, and Hall compared the benefits to schizophrenic patients of an individual-centered activity (called traditional occupational therapy) and a group-centered activity (making lawn chairs for the hospital). They found no significant difference in benefits between the activities. They found, "However, there is some support for the hypothesis that, for the activities studied, the personality of the therapist is more important than the activity per se" (p. 123/555). Like earlier studies of occupational therapy group treatment, this investigation was not conducted by occupational therapists but by three male therapists in a Veterans Administration Hospital (a PhD, an MD, and an EdM).

The increased use of group treatment in the 1950s resulted from several factors (Box 2-16). After World War II, many veterans needed psychiatric treatment to help them readjust to peacetime. With the availability of medication to control behavior, therapists could design groups to help patients move from hospital life to community living (Feuss and Maltby, 1959; Moss and Stewart, 1959). It is not coincidental that occupational therapists, many of whom were employed by the army, applied concepts from the growing field of group dynamics to their practice. Another factor was the interest of social scientists in studying small group behavior (Mosey, 1971). Four major studies on the use of occupational therapy group treatment for community adjustment of psychotic patients were conducted in Veterans Administration Hospitals during the 1950s (Bobis, Harrison, and Traub, 1955; Efron, Marks, and Hall, 1959; Levine, Marks, and Hall, 1957; Nelson et al., 1956).

Many therapists in the 1950s were more prepared to apply theoretical material to their practice, a result of several schools' standards that required an undergraduate degree prior to admission into an occupational therapy certificate program (Jantzen, 1972).

Box 2-16
Increased Understanding

Mosey (1971) attributed the changes that occurred in this period to the following developments: occupational therapists' more sophisticated understanding of specific diseases, the development of psychiatric theories that viewed problematic interpersonal relationships as the cause of mental illness, the use of a team approach and medication in the care of psychiatric patients, and the new theoretical perspective of social scientists who were studying small groups.

Ego Building–Psychodynamic Era: 1962–1969

By the end of the 1950s, occupational therapy, just as other life sciences, had shifted its focus from a holistic to a reductionist paradigm (Kielhofner and Burke, 1977). This shift resulted from medicine's attempt to achieve scientific status by becoming more like physical science and its subsequent pressuring of occupational therapy to accept a reductionist model as well (Kielhofner and Burke, 1977).

The emphasis on group dynamics and process in occupational therapy group treatment was different from the technical view of patients and treatment emerging in the 1950s. However, the growth of reductionism in other areas of occupational therapy and in medicine was more influential than the trend toward more holistic occupational therapy group approaches. With the growth of a holistic perspective in group treatment, one may wonder if occupational therapists who led groups were different from their professional counterparts who did not lead groups. Regardless, given the historically subordinate position of all occupational therapists, this scenario was predictable. According to Kielhofner and Burke (1977), "By the end of the 1950s, the reductionist model was brought into occupational therapy as the basis of a new paradigm" (p. 682). The reductionist paradigm, they observed, took three forms: (1) the kinesiological model; (2) the psychoanalytic, or interpersonal communication, model; and (3) the sensory integrative, or neurological, model. The three models reflected the attempt to establish a scientific basis for practice.

These forms of a single paradigm are termed reductionist because of the single goal they share. Therapists attempted to define more narrowly the specific goals to be achieved and to achieve them in a more direct manner. Therapists attempted to help patients explore the intrapsychic determinants, or psychodynamics, of their maladaptive behavior through a task-oriented group. The growth of the 1950s was now strictly channeled to achieve specific ends (Box 2-17).

The 1960s was also an era of change in many other areas. Diasio (1971) summarized crises that had major social impact: the Vietnam War, urban riots, planned obsolescence, campus unrest, rising crime, inflation, and environmental pollution. Balanced against these crises were the more positive trends of the consumer protection movements, peace and civil rights movements, women's liberation movements, concern for the ecology and community health pro-

---

Box 2-17
Building Abilities

The occupational therapy group was often aimed at developing ego strengths: the patient's ability to test reality, apply judgment, make decisions, and modify behavior on the basis of self-observation.

grams, the desire for community control, and the human potential movement (Diasio, 1971). These social crises and movements, in turn, affected group treatment. Like other professionals, occupational therapists perceived the need for social and scientific accountability.

Research in this period reflected the growing awareness of the need for long-term concern. In their dynamic "four-phase concept" approach, Linn, Weinroth, and Shamah (1962) suggested that the occupational therapist provide an "unstructured work situation" so that changes in the patient's psychiatric illness could be detected. They, two physicians and an occupational therapist, hypothesized that the patient hospitalized for an acute psychiatric illness progressed through four distinct phases: (1) acute emotional decompensation, (2) initial emotional restitution, (3) predischarge symptom flare-up, and (4) meaning reaction (following discharge from inpatient treatment). This concept of group treatment followed trends in hospital psychiatry.

Fidler (1966) described the prototype for occupational therapy group treatment in the psychodynamic era of the 1960s:

> These groups are structured for the purpose of providing a group experience wherein members may explore the many and varied problems which arise in the process of task selection and completion such as decision making, accepting responsibility, being productive, and sharing with others. Individual feelings and behavior are discussed in terms of how they impede or enhance group cohesiveness and task accomplishment. (p. 73)

This approach supported the concept of milieu therapy. Material brought up in occupational therapy groups was then discussed in verbal psychotherapy and other individual and group therapies.

As the research just described indicates, occupational therapy groups were guided by two fundamental principles during the psychodynamic period. First, if exposed to a healthy milieu of accepting and cooperative staff and a variety of self-initiated activities with a range of emotional-interpersonal demands, the patient will develop or reconstitute ego skills necessary for community living (Barker and Muir, 1969; Fidler and Fidler, 1963; German, 1964; Lamb, 1967; Llorens, 1968; Llorens and Johnson, 1966; Llorens and Rubin, 1967; Reilly, 1966; Shannon and Snortum, 1965; Slavson, 1967/1979). Second, if given an interpersonal task in a group, opportunity for the group to develop into a cohesive unit, feedback on the nature of interactions, and modeling of appropriate social skills or responses, the patient can develop ego skills for adapting to interpersonal situations (Fidler, 1966, 1969; Gillette and Mayer, 1968; Howe, 1968; Johnston, 1965; Mosey, 1968, 1969; Owen and Newman, 1965; Rothaus, Hanson, and Cleveland, 1966; Shannon and Snortum, 1965). The goals and methods of occupational therapy groups thus became in part like those of psychotherapy groups (Box 2-18).

The 1960s were a hallmark period for occupational therapy group treatment. Many papers describing occupational therapy group formats were written during this period, and group work flourished as a form of treatment. The concern for a scientific approach was exemplified by the many empirical papers on

> **Box 2-18**
> **Opening Doors**
>
> Through occupational therapy groups, individuals found healthy modes of self-expression, gained improved self-esteem, and found emotional satisfaction of their needs.

occupational therapy group treatment. Several studies focused on the effectiveness of activity groups for promoting social interaction (Ellsworth and Colman, 1969; Gralewicz, Hill, and Mackinson, 1968; Pasework and Hornby, 1968; Pearman and Newman, 1968; Werner, Maddigan, and Watson, 1969). The American Occupational Therapy Association responded to its membership's need for a more sophisticated understanding of evaluation methods, treatment planning, and treatment of psychiatric patients (Mazer, 1968). In an attempt to encourage participation in the newly developing community mental health programs and to improve professional training in the treatment of psychiatric patients, the Association conducted national and regional educational institutes from 1964 through 1968. These seminars supported the psychiatrists' dynamic model of group psychotherapy and adapted it to occupational therapy by introducing an activity process into the group (Gillette and Mayer, 1968) (Box 2-19).

Adaptation Era: 1970s–1990s

The reductionist trend of the 1960s did not last beyond the decade and ultimately left many occupational therapists dissatisfied with their roles as therapists. Kielhofner and Burke (1977) speculated that in the 1960s occupational therapists were concerned with the inadequacy of their theoretical knowledge and were confused about their roles as health professionals. The two researchers surmised, "The problems of social adaptation, for which the medical model was inadequate and which was not addressed by reductionism, are anomalies that earmarked the failure of reductionism in the clinical arena of occupational therapy" (p. 685).

The advances of medical research in developing drugs to treat a wide range of mental illnesses and expanding our understanding of biological and chemical processes did not resolve the problems of living in the world for people cop-

> **Box 2-19**
> **Filling a Need**
>
> In the late 1960s, occupational therapists once again responded to the external pressures of the medical community, as well as to the growing social concerns and needs of the general public.

Box 2-20
Focus on Adaptation

In the 1970s and 1980s the literature on occupational therapy groups focused on problems of adaptation.

ing with day-to-day life. As more types of patients were defined, the limits of medicine—strictly defined—came to be recognized. Medical treatment could not aid the chronically disabled, nonverbal, or noninsightful to cope with living among other people. As practitioners in the field of occupational therapy came to recognize the types of problems still unsolved, they sought forms of group therapy that would address these problems (Box 2-20). The groups described in the literature of the 1970s and 1980s were designed to help patients meet their health needs, cope with skill deficiencies, overcome performance problems, and manage environmental constraints.

The newly developing goals and concerns of the profession were reinforced by external economic factors. During the 1970s, the U.S. economy faced a severe recession, which led to restricted funding, reduced hospital stays, increased demand for quality assurance, and improved cost/benefit ratios. The Bureau of Labor Statistics of the United States Department of Labor predicted a "substantial shortfall of occupational therapy personnel" through 1990 (Acquaviva and Presseller, 1983, p. 79). According to Acquaviva and Presseller (1983):

> over the past 15 to 20 years we have seen rapid growth in supply of personnel, with a concurrent rapid expansion of the demand for occupational therapy services, resulting in an overall shortage of personnel (Box 2-21). That shortage has become more acute in the late 1970s and early '80s at a time when our ability to satisfy that shortage is diminishing. The ramifications of this situation are very serious. (pp. 79–80)

Group treatment flourished in the economic climate of the 1970s. Given the need for serving large numbers of patients at a reduced or maintained cost with fewer personnel, the need for occupational therapy group treatment grew in the 1980s.

The number of occupational therapists enrolled in an accredited entry-level

Box 2-21
Mirroring Society

Along with the demands for more efficient and economical services, occupational therapy faced an extensive shortage of trained personnel between 1970 and 1981.

> **Box 2-22**
> **Groups Flourish**
>
> Group treatment was viewed in many situations as a preferred treatment by practitioners, as well as promoted and implemented by these same therapists in their careers as administrators.

master's program increased dramatically. In 1970, for example, 142 students were enrolled in such programs; by 1981, 577 students were enrolled (Dataline, 1982). These students were trained in the use of groups as a treatment modality since the 1970s (Delworth, 1972; "Essentials of an Accredited Educational Program for the Occupational Therapist," 1975; Maynard and Pedro, 1971; Posthuma and Posthuma, 1972). The importance of group dynamics, self-awareness, and the interdisciplinary team were also stressed in occupational therapy curricula and practice (Odhner, 1970b; Steiner, 1972).

The educational trends of the 1970s were followed by an increase in the use of groups in the 1980s (Box 2-22). The direction of the theoretical work of that period was signaled by Ellsworth and Colman (1969), who proposed that treatment be based on behavior principles, specifically, the behavioral approach of B. F. Skinner, which stresses reinforcement and reward for desired behavior. This theoretical approach allowed therapists to concentrate on helping patients adapt their behavior to situational needs and goals (Box 2-23). Occupational therapy groups in this period focused on the patients' skill deficits (Denton, 1982; Fidler, 1984; Goldstein, Gershaw, and Spraflin, 1979; Hersen and Luber, 1977; Hughes and Mullins, 1981; Kramer and Beidel, 1982; Maslen, 1982; Mosey, 1970a, 1970b, 1981; Neistadt and Marques, 1984; Stein, 1982; Talbot, 1983) and social well-being (Mosey, 1973a, 1973b, 1974).

Occupational therapy groups of the Adaptation Era were generally based on one of three factors (Box 2-24): (1) diagnosis, (2) role, or (3) setting. Groups based on diagnosis include the following:

hemiplegic exercise groups (Bouchard, 1972)

stroke groups (Wilson, 1979)

emotion groups (Angel, 1981)

> **Box 2-23**
> **Adaptable Treatments**
>
> Whether the group was for treatment of a physical problem or an emotional one, the emphasis seemed to be on social adaptation through structured, graded learning experiences.

Box 2-24
Groups Classified

During the Adaptation Era, occupational therapy groups were usually grouped according to one of three types:

Diagnosis

Hemiplegia

Stroke

Emotion

Hyperactive/learning disabled children

Parkinson's

Spinal cord injury

Alcoholism

Regressed/elderly psychiatric

Schizophrenic/borderline patients

Arthritic ROM

Roles

Physically disabled

Women

Elderly/Adolescent psychiatric

Children with emotional disorders and psychiatric patients in the community

Occupational Therapy students

Occupational Therapists returning to the job market

Setting

Acute care facilities

Psychiatric outpatient clinics

Extended care facilities

Community elderly

Geriatric day hospitals

Emergency psychiatric

groups for hyperactive and learning disabled children (Cermak, Stein, and Abelson, 1973; McKibbin and King, 1983)

Parkinson's groups (Gauthier, Daziel, Gauthier, 1987)

spinal cord injury groups (Mann, Godfrey, and Dowd, 1973)

alcoholism groups (Lindsay, 1983)

groups for regressed and elderly psychiatric patients (Noce, Breuninger, and Noce, 1983; Ross and Burdick, 1978)

patients with schizophrena (King, 1974; Linn et al., 1979; Odhner, 1970a; VanderRoest and Clements, 1983)

borderline patients (Goodman, 1983)

arthritis range of motion (ROM) groups

Groups focusing on roles deal with the following:

physically disabled (Versluys, 1980)

women (Donohue, 1982)

elderly and adolescent psychiatric patients (Mahier and Tachabrun, 1978)

children with emotional disorders (Fahl, 1970)

psychiatric patients in the community (Broekema, Danz, and Schloemer, 1975; Heine, 1975; Webb, 1973)

groups for occupational therapy students (Botkins, 1979) and occupational therapists returning to the job market (Labovitz, 1978)

Groups concerned with the setting include the following:

groups for acute care facilities (Corry, Sebastian, and Mosey, 1974; Neville, 1980)

psychiatric outpatient clinics (Kuenstler, 1976)

extended care facilities (Fearing, 1978)

community elderly (Menks, Sittles, Weaver, and Yanow, 1977)

geriatric day hospitals (Aronson, 1976; Kiernat, 1976)

emergency psychiatric settings (Hyman and Metzker, 1970)

The unifying thread in these groups was their concern for helping the patient develop daily living skills and function through adaptation.

Toward the end of the 1980s, an increasing number of occupational therapists were employed in school systems to work with children who have special needs. Goals of treatment were more for habilitation and prevention than for rehabilitation. Service delivery followed a community model rather than the medical model. Policies in school systems varied from community to community. In some schools, children could be treated in small groups; in others, occupational therapy was done only on a one-to-one basis.

With the increased economic pressures on medical care, more attention was given to documenting the cost effectiveness of group treatment as compared to individual treatment (Gauthier, Daziel, and Gauthier, 1987; Kurasik, 1967; Trahey, 1991). Increased hospital costs, the movement of patients to community programs, and home treatment have necessitated a skills-oriented, outcome-focused approach to groups, as well as group leaders, who often work as facilitators, consultants, and educators to informal groups in the community.

The group approach to treatment became the most economical for both the patient and the service delivery system. Increased hospital costs and the movement of patients into community programs necessitated a behavioral, skills-oriented learning approach, and this quickly became the paradigm for occupational therapy groups.

Conclusion

The adaptation approach of the 1970s and 1980s echoed the introduction of occupational therapy groups in the 1920s; in fact, there were many reports of activity-focused groups in the Adaptation Era (Falk-Kessler and Froschauer, 1978; Fearing, 1978; Goldstein and Collins, 1982; Kiernat, 1979; Rance and Price, 1973; Rider and Gramlin, 1980; Schuman, Marcus, and Nesse, 1973; Schwartzberg, Howe, and McDermott, 1982). These contemporary groups, however, were only superficially like the early groups in 1922. In the Adaptation Era, groups clearly had a functional aim and a theoretical rationale. Socialization and communication were always goals, as was the use of activity to increase physical, cognitive, social, or task skills.

In the Project Era, the early form of the occupational therapy group was described as a collective. This was an organized unit although it did not necessarily have a unified goal or an interdependent task like the group-centered unit. By the 1970s, the Adaptation Era, the group format was determined according to specific factors related to the patients, as well as the type of reimbursement and staffing available. Today, patients' skill deficits, degrees of social well-being, diagnoses, and role problems are considered when groups are formed in an occupational therapy program. Finally, the conceptual model and theoretical orientation are now regularly considered in choosing the format of a group. For example, in a long-term program with a behavioral orientation, patients with minimal self-care skills are often placed in a parallel, didactic skills learning group similar to the collective. For higher functioning patients in an acute care program with a biopsychosocial orientation, occupational therapy might take a more interdependent group approach and stress self-awareness through group self-expression activities.

The occupational therapist of the 1980s was also different from the therapist of the Project Era (Box 2-25). Women moved into the mainstream of work in America and demanded more formal higher education. As a result, occupa-

Box 2-25
Defining Change

Although women have dominated occupational therapy throughout its history, the definition of the therapist changed in the 1980s.

tional therapists are now better educated and are drawn from more varied socioeconomic backgrounds.

Even as its form has changed through the years, professionals remain convinced of the value of the occupational therapy group as a treatment tool. Occupational therapy groups have provided service to many patients, often in times of severe economic crisis in the United States. This explains in part why they have been so important to therapists, patients, and physicians. During the next few decades, we can expect a deeper understanding of the curative, as well as rehabilitative, effects of occupational therapy group treatment, and a growing interest in its use.

Review Questions

1. How did the occupational therapy groups in the Project Era differ from those in the Group Dynamics–Process Era? Name some of the events that are responsible for these differences. Did the role of the group activity change?
2. How do economic conditions affect the use of group treatment in occupational therapy programs? Give examples.
3. How did the group dynamics movement of the Process Era change the ways that group treatment was organized? How did the occupational therapist's role as a group leader change?
4. Throughout the history of occupational therapy group treatment, changes have occurred in response to influences in medical practice and economic pressures. Describe some of these influences and the changes they generated.

References

Acquaviva, F. A., and Presseller, S. (1983). Nationally speaking: Occupational therapy manpower. American Journal of Occupational Therapy 37(2): 79–81.

American Occupational Therapy Association (1955). Institute: Theme interpersonal relationships. American Journal of Occupational Therapy 9(5): (Part II) 212–223, 230–232.

Anderson, C. L. (1936). Project work: An individualized group therapy. Occupational Therapy and Rehabilitation 15(4): 265–269.

Angel, S. L. (1981). The emotion identification group. American Journal of Occupational Therapy 35(4): 256–262.

Aronson, R. (1976). The role of an occupational therapist in a geriatric day hospital setting—Maimonides Day Hospital. American Journal of Occupational Therapy 30(5): 290–292.

Barker, P., and Muir, A. M. (1969). The role of occupational therapy in a children's inpatient psychiatric unit. American Journal of Occupational Therapy, 23(5): 431–436.

Bing, R. K. (1981). Eleanor Clarke Slagle Lectureship—1981. Occupational therapy revisited: A paraphrastic journey. American Journal of Occupational Therapy 35(8): 499–518.

Blackman, N. (1940). Experiences with a literary club in the group treatment of schizophrenia. Occupational Therapy and Rehabilitation 19(5): 293–303.

Bobis, B. R., Harrison, R. M., and Traub, L. (1955). Activity group therapy. American Journal of Occupational Therapy 9(1): 19–21, 50.

Bockoven, J. S. (1971). Occupational therapy—A historic perspective. Legacy of moral treatment—1800s to 1910. American Journal of Occupational Therapy 25(5): 223–225.

Botkins, S. (1979). A peer discussion group of senior occupational therapy students. American Journal of Occupational Therapy 33(2): 123–125.

Bouchard, V. C. (1972). Hemiplegic exercise and discussion group. American Journal of Occupational Therapy 26(7): 330–331.

Broekema, M. C., Danz, K. H., and Schloemer, C. U. (1975). Occupational therapy in a community aftercare program. American Journal of Occupational Therapy 29(1): 22–27.

Canton, E. L. (1923). Psychology of occupational therapy. Archives of Occupational Therapy 2(5): 347–357.

Cermak, S. A., Stein, F., and Abelson, C. (1973). Hyperactive children and an activity group therapy model. American Journal of Occupational Therapy 26(6): 311–315.

Chafe, W. H. (1972). The American Woman: Her Changing Social, Economic, and Political Roles, 1920–1970. New York: Oxford University Press.

Combs, M. H. (1959). An activities program in a custodial care group. American Journal of Occupational Therapy 13(1): 5–8, 26–27.

Corry, S., Sebastian, V., and Mosey, A. C. (1974). Acute short-term treatment in psychiatry. American Journal of Occupational Therapy 28(7): 401–406.

Dataline (1982). Occupational Therapy Newspaper 36(11): 3.

Delworth, U. M. (1972). Interpersonal skill development for occupational therapy students. American Journal of Occupational Therapy 26(1): 27–29.

Denton, P. L. (1982). Teaching interpersonal skills with videotape. Occupational Therapy in Mental Health: A Journal of Psychosocial Practice and Research 2(4): 17–33.

Diasio, K. (1971). Occupational therapy—A historical perspective: The modern era—1960 to 1970. American Journal of Occupational Therapy 25(5): 237–242.

Donohue, M. V. (1982). Designing activities to develop a women's identification group. Occupational Therapy in Mental Health: A Journal of Psychosocial Practice and Research 2(1): 1–19.

Dunton, W. R. (1937). Quilt making as a socializing measure. Occupational Therapy and Rehabilitation 16(4): 275–278.

Efron, H. Y., Marks, H. K., and Hall, R. (1959). A comparison of group-centered and individual-centered activity programs. Archives of General Psychiatry 1(5): 120/552–123/555.

Ellsworth, P. D., and Colman, A. D. (1969). A model program: The application of operant conditioning principles to work group experience. American Journal of Occupational Therapy 23(6): 495–501.

Essentials of an accredited educational program for the occupational therapist. (1975). Established and adopted by the American Occupational Therapy Association, Inc. Council on Education October 1972 in collaboration with the American Medical Association Council on Medical Education. Adopted by the American Medical Association House of Delegates, June 1973. American Journal of Occupational Therapy 29(8): 485–496.

Fahl, M. A. (1970). Emotionally disturbed children: Effects of cooperative and competitive activity on peer interaction. American Journal of Occupational Therapy 24(1): 31–33.

Falk-Kessler, J., and Froschauer, K. H. (1978). The soap opera: A dynamic group approach for psychiatric patients. American Journal of Occupational Therapy 32(5): 317–319.

Fearing, V. G. (1978). An authors group for extended care patients. American Journal of Occupational Therapy 32(8): 526–527.

Feuss, C. D., and Maltby, J. W. (1959). Occupational therapy in the community. American Journal of Occupational Therapy 13(1): 9–10, 25.

Fidler, G. S. (1966). A second look at work as a primary force in rehabilitation and treatment. American Journal of Occupational Therapy 20(2): 72–74.

Fidler, G. S. (1969). The task-oriented group as a context for treatment. American Journal of Occupational Therapy 23(1): 43–48.

Fidler, G. S. (1984). Design of Rehabilitation Services in Psychiatric Hospital Settings. Laurel, MD: Ramsco.

Fidler, G. S., and Fidler, J. W. (1954). Introduction to Psychiatric Occupational Therapy. New York: MacMillan.

Fidler, G. S., and Fidler, J. W. (1960). Introduction to Psychiatric Occupational Therapy (2nd ed.). New York: MacMillan.

Fidler, G. S., and Fidler, J. W. (1963). Occupational Therapy: A Communication Process in Psychiatry. New York: MacMillan.

Gauthier, L., Dalziel, S. and Gauthier, S. (1987). The benefits of group occupational therapy for patients with Parkinson's disease. American Journal of Occupational Therapy, 41: 360–365.

German, S. A. (1964). A group approach to rehabilitation occupational therapy in a psychiatric setting. American Journal of Occupational Therapy 18(5): 209–214.

Gibb, J. R. (1958). The occupational therapist works with groups. American Journal of Occupational Therapy 12(4): 205–214.

Gillette, N., and Kielhofner, G. (1979). The impact of specialization on the professionalization and survival of occupational therapy. American Journal of Occupational Therapy 33(1): 20–28.

Gillette, N. P., and Mayer, P. R. (1968). The group method in occupational therapy. In J. L. Mazer (Project Director), Final Report Rehabilitation Services Administration Grant Number 123-T-68 for Field Consultant in Psychiatric Rehabilitation. New York: American Occupational Therapy Association.

Gleave, G. M. (1947). Occupational therapy in children's hospitals and pediatric services. In H. S. Willard and C. S. Spackman (eds.), Principles of Occupational Therapy. Philadelphia: J. B. Lippincott.

Goldstein, A. P., Gershaw, N. J., and Spraflin, R. P. (1979). Structured learning therapy: Development and evaluation. American Journal of Occupational Therapy 33(10): 635–639.

Goldstein, N., and Collins, T. (1982). Making videotapes: An activity for hospitalized adolescents. American Journal of Occupational Therapy 36(8): 530–533.

Goodman, G. B. (1983). Occupational therapy treatment: Interventions with borderline patients. Occupational Therapy in Mental Health: A Journal of Psychosocial Practice and Research 3(3): 19–31.

Gralewicz, A., Hill, B., and Mackinson, M. (1968). Restoration therapy: An approach to group therapy for the chronically ill. American Journal of Occupation Therapy 22(4): 294–299.

Gratke, B. E., and Lux, P. A. (1960). Psychiatric occupational therapy in a milieu setting. American Journal of Occupational Therapy 14(1): 13–16.

Halle, L., and Landy, A. (1948). The integration of group activity and group therapy. Occupational Therapy and Rehabilitation 27(4): 286–298.

Heine, D. B. (1975). Daily living group: Focus on transition from hospital to community. American Journal of Occupational Therapy 29(10): 628–630.

Hersen, M., and Luber, R. F. (1977). Use of group psychotherapy in a partial hospitalization service: The remediation of basic skill deficits. International Journal of Group Psychotherapy 27(3): 361–376.

Hopkins, H. L. (1978). An historical perspective on occupational therapy. In H. L. Hopkins and H. D. Smith (eds.), Willard and Spackman's Occupational Therapy (5th ed.). Philadelphia: J. B. Lippincott, pp. 3–23.

Howe, M. C. (1968). An occupational therapy activity group. American Journal of Occupational Therapy 22(3): 176–179.

Hughes, P. L., and Mullins, L. (1981). Acute Psychiatric Care: An Occupational Therapy Guide to Exercises in Daily Living Skills. Thorofare, NJ: Charles B. Slack.

Hyde, R. W., York, R., and Wood, A. C. (1948). Effectiveness of games in a mental hospital. Occupational Therapy and Rehabilitation 27(4): 304–308.

Hyman, M., and Metzker, J. R. (1970). Occupational therapy in an emergency psychiatric setting. American Journal of Occupational Therapy 24(4): 280–283.

Jantzen, A. C. (1972). Some characteristics of female occupational therapists, 1970, Part III: A comparison: Faculty and clinical practitioners. American Journal of Occupational Therapy 26(3): 150–154.

Johnston, N. (1965). Group reading as a treatment tool with geriatrics. American Journal of Occupational Therapy 19(4): 192–195.

Kielhofner, G., and Burke, J. P. (1977). Occupational therapy after 60 years: An account of changing identity and knowledge. American Journal of Occupational Therapy 31(10): 674–689.

Kiernat, J. M. (1976). Geriatric day hospitals: A golden opportunity for therapists. American Journal of Occupational Therapy 30(5): 285–289.

Kiernat, J. M. (1979). The use of life review activity with confused nursing home residents. American Journal of Occupational Therapy 33(5): 306–310.

King, L. J. (1974). A sensory-integrative approach to schizophrenia. American Journal of Occupational Therapy 28(9): 529–536.

Koven, B., and Shuff, F. L. (1953). Group therapy with the chronically ill. American Journal of Occupational Therapy 7(5): 208–209, 219.

Kramer, L. W., and Beidel, D. C. (1982). Job seeking skills groups: A review and application to a chronic psychiatric population. Occupational Therapy in Mental Health: A Journal of Psychosocial Practice and Research 2(2): 37–44.

Kuenstler, G. (1976). A planning group for psychiatric outpatients. American Journal of Occupational Therapy 30(10): 634–639.

Kurasik, S. (1967). Group dynamics in rehabilitation of hemiplegic patients. Journal of the American Geriatic Society 15: 852–855.

Labovitz, D. R. (1978). The returning therapist: A group approach. American Journal of Occupational Therapy 32(9): 580–585.

Lakin, M., and Dray, M. (1958). Psychological aspects of activity for the aged. American Journal of Occupational Therapy 12(4): 172–175, 187–188.

Lamb, R. H. (1967). Chronic psychiatric patients in the day hospital. Archives of General Psychiatry 17: 615–621.

Leuret, F. (1840/1948). On the moral treatment of insanity. In S. Licht (ed. and trans.), Occupational Therapy Source Book. Baltimore: Williams & Wilkins. (Article originally written in 1840.)

Levine, D., Marks, H. K., and Hall, R. (1957). Differential effect of factors in an activity therapy program. American Journal of Psychiatry 114: 532–535.

Licht, S. (ed.) (1948). Occupational Therapy Source Book. Baltimore: Williams & Wilkins.

Lindsay, W. P. (1983). The role of the occupational therapist in treatment of alcoholism. American Journal of Occupational Therapy 37(1): 36–43.

Linn, L., Weinroth, M. D., and Shamah, R. (1962). Occupational Therapy in Dynamic Psychiatry: An Introduction to the Four-Phase Concept in Hospital Psychiatry. Washington, DC: The American Psychiatric Association.

Linn, M. W., Caffey, E. M., Klett, C. J., Hogarty, G. E., and Lamb, H. R. (1979). Day treatment and psychotropic drugs in the aftercare of schizophrenic patients. Archives of General Psychiatry 36: 1055–1066.

Llorens, L. A. (1968). Changing methods in treatment of psychosocial dysfunction. American Journal of Occupational Therapy 22(1): 26–29.

Llorens, L. A., and Johnson, P. A. (1966). Occupational therapy in an ego-oriented milieu. American Journal of Occupational Therapy 20(4): 178–181.

Llorens, L. A., and Rubin, E. Z. (1967). Developing Ego Functions in Disturbed Children: Occupational Therapy in Milieu. Detroit: Wayne State University Press.

Lockerbie, L., and Stevenson, G. H. (1947). Socialization through occupational therapy. Occupational Therapy and Rehabilitation 26(3): 142–145.

Mahier, S. H., and Tachabrun, B. R. (1978). Experience and youth group: For elderly and adolescent psychiatric patients. American Journal of Occupational Therapy 32(2): 115–117.

Mann, W., Godfrey, M. E., and Dowd, E. T. (1973). The use of group counseling procedures in the rehabilitation of spinal cord injured patients. American Journal of Occupational Therapy 27(2): 73–77.

Markowitz, G. E., and Rosner, D. (1979). Doctors in crisis: Medical education and medical reform during the progressive era, 1895–1915. In S. Reverby and D. Rosner (eds.), Health Care in America: Essays in Social History. Philadelphia: Temple University Press.

Marsh, L. C. (1936). Group treatment of relatives of psychotic patients. Occupational Therapy and Rehabilitation 15(1): 1–17.

Maslen, D. (1982). Rehabilitation training for community living skills: Concepts and techniques. Occupational Therapy in Mental Health: A Journal of Psychosocial Practice and Research 2(1): 33–49.

Maynard, M., and Pedro, D. (1971). One day experience in group dynamics in an occupational therapy assistant course. American Journal of Occupational Therapy 25(3): 170–171.

Mazer, J. L. (Project Director) (1968). Final Report Rehabilitation Services Administration Grant Number 123-T-68 for Field Consultant in Psychiatric Rehabilitation. New York: American Occupational Therapy Association.

McKibbin, E., and King, J. (1983). Activity group counseling for learning-disabled children with behavior problems. American Journal of Occupational Therapy 37(9): 617–623.

Menks, F., Sittles, S., Weaver, D., and Yanow, B. (1977). A psychogeriatric activity group in a rural community. American Journal of Occupational Therapy 31(6): 376–384.

Meyer, A. (1922/1977). The philosophy of occupational therapy. American Journal of Occupational Therapy 31(10): 639–642. (Originally published 1922.)

Mosey, A. C. (1968). Recapitulation of ontogenesis: A theory for practice of occupational therapy. American Journal of Occupational Therapy 22(5): 426–432.

Mosey, A. C. (1969). Dependency and integrative skill as they relate to affinity for and acceptance by an assigned group. American Journal of Occupational Therapy 23(4): 348–349.

Mosey, A. C. (1970a). The concept and use of developmental groups. American Journal of Occupational Therapy 24(4): 272–275.

Mosey, A. C. (1970b). Three Frames of Reference for Mental Health. Thorofare, NJ: Charles B. Slack.

Mosey, A. C. (1971). Occupational therapy: A historical perspective. Involvement in the rehabilitation movement—1942–1960. American Journal of Occupational Therapy 25(5): 234–236.

Mosey, A. C. (1973a). Activities Therapy. New York: Raven Press.

Mosey, A. C. (1973b). Meeting health needs. American Journal of Occupational Therapy 27(1): 14–17.

Mosey, A. C. (1974). An alternative: The biopsychosocial model. American Journal of Occupational Therapy 28(3): 137–140.

Mosey, A. C. (1981). Occupational Therapy: Configuration of a Profession. New York: Raven Press.

Moss, F. B., and Stewart, G. (1959). A program for geriatric patients from hospital to community. American Journal of Occupational Therapy 13(6): 268–271.

Neistadt, M. E., and Marques, K. (1984). An independent living skills training program. American Journal of Occupational Therapy 38(10): 671–676.

Nelson, A., Mackenthun, D., Bloesch, M., Milan, A., Unrein, M., and Hill, K. (1956). A preliminary report on a study in group occupational therapy. American Journal of Occupational Therapy 10(5): 254–258, 262–263, 271.

Neville, A. (1980). Temporal adaptation: Application with short-term psychiatric patients. American Journal of Occupational Therapy 34(5): 328–331.

Noce, S. F., Breuninger, P. L., and Noce, J. S. (1983). A Piagetian-based approach for the assessment and occupational therapy treatment of cognitive deficits in process schizophrenic and psychogeriatric patients. In W. E. Kelly (ed.), The Changing Role of Rehabilitation Medicine in the Management of the Psychiatric Patient. Springfield, IL: Charles C. Thomas, pp. 107–121.

Novick, L. J. (1961). Occupational therapy and social group work in the home for the sick aged: A comparison. American Journal of Occupational Therapy 15(5): 198–203, 211.

Odhner, F. (1970a). A study of group tasks as facilitators of verbalization among hospitalized schizophrenic patients. American Journal of Occupational Therapy 24(1): 7–12.

Odhner, F. (1970b). Group dynamics of the interdisciplinary team. American Journal of Occupational Therapy 24(7): 484–487.

Owen, C., and Newman, N. (1965). Utilizing films as a therapeutic agent in group interaction. American Journal of Occupational Therapy 19(4): 205–207.

Pasework, R. and Hornby, R. (1968). The effect upon social interaction patterns of a short-term stimulation program for psychiatric geriatric patients. American Journal of Occupational Therapy 22(3): 195–196.

Pearman, H. E., and Newman, N. (1968). Work-oriented occupational therapy for the geriatric patient. American Journal of Occupational Therapy 22(3): 203–208.

Posthuma, B. W. and Posthuma, A. B. (1972). The effect of a small-group experience on occupational therapy students. American Journal of Occupational Therapy 26(8): 415–418.

Rance, C., and Price, A. (1973). Poetry as a group project. American Journal of Occupational Therapy 27(5): 252–255.

Reed, K. L., and Sanderson, S. R. (1980). Concepts of Occupational Therapy. Baltimore: Williams & Wilkins.

Reilly, M. (1966). A psychiatric occupational therapy program as a teaching model. American Journal of Occupational Therapy 20(2): 61–67.

Rerek, M. D. (1971). Occupational therapy: A historical perspective. The Depression years— 1929 to 1941. American Journal of Occupational Therapy 25(5): 231–233.

Rider, B. B. and Gramlin, J. T. (1980). An activities approach to occupational therapy in a short-term acute mental health unit. American Occupational Therapy Association Mental Health Specialty Section Newsletter 3(4): Rockville, MD.

Rosner, D. (1979). Business at the bedside: Health care in Brooklyn, 1890–1915. In S. Reverby and D. Rosner (eds.), Health Care in America: Essays in Social History. Philadelphia: Temple University Press.

Ross, M., and Burdick, D. (1978). A Sensory Integration Training Manual for Regressed and Geriatric Patients. Middletown, CT: Department of Rehabilitation Services, Connecticut Valley Hospital.

Rothaus, P., Hanson, P. G., and Cleveland, S. E. (1966). Art and group dynamics. American Journal of Occupational Therapy 20(4): 182–187.

Rothman, D. J. (1980). Conscience and Convenience: The Asylum and its Alternatives in Progressive America. Boston: Little, Brown & Company.

Schiffer, M. (1979). The genealogy of group psychotherapy. In S. R. Slavson (author) and M. Schiffer (ed.), Dynamics of Group Psychotherapy. New York: Jason Aronson.

Schuman, S. H., Marcus, D., and Nesse, D. (1973). Puppetry and the mentally ill. American Journal of Occupational Therapy 27(8): 484–486.

Schwartzberg, S. L., Howe, M. C., and McDermott, A. (1982). Comparison of three treatment group formats for facilitating social interaction. Occupational Therapy in Mental Health: A Journal of Psychosocial Practice and Research 2(4): 1–16.

Shannon, P. D., and Snortum, J. R., (1965). An activity group's role in intensive psychotherapy. American Journal of Occupational Therapy 19(6): 344–347.

Slagle, E. C. (1922). Training aides for mental patients. Archives of Occupational Therapy 1(1): 11–17.

Slavson, S. R. (1979). Vita-Erg therapy with long-term, regressed psychotic women. In S. R. Slavson (author) and M. Schiffer (ed.), Dynamics of Group Psychotherapy. New York: Jason Aronson. (Article originally written in 1967.)

Smuts, R. W. (1959). Women and Work in America. New York: Columbia University Press.

Solomon, A. P., and Fentress, T. L. (1947). A critical study of analytically oriented group psychotherapy utilizing the technique of dramatization of the psychodynamics. Occupational Therapy and Rehabilitation 26(1): 23–46.

Springfield, F. B., and Tullis, L. H. (1958). An intensive activities program for chronic neuropsychiatric patients. American Journal of Occupational Therapy 12(5): 247–249.

Stein, F. (1982). A current review of the behavioral frame of reference and its application to occupational therapy. Occupational Therapy in Mental Health: A Journal of Psychosocial Practice and Research 2(4): 35–62.

Steiner, J. (1972). Reflections on the encounter group and the therapist. American Journal of Occupational Therapy 26(3): 130–131.

Talbot, J. F. (1983). An inpatient adolescent living skills program. Occupational Therapy in Mental Health: A Journal of Psychosocial Practice and Research 3(4): 35–45.

Trahey, P. J. (1991). A comparison of the cost-effectiveness of two types of occupational therapy services. American Journal of Occupational Therapy 45: 397–401.

VanderRoest, L. L., and Clements, S. T. (1983). Sensory Integration: Rationale and Treatment Activities for Groups. Grand Rapids, MI: South Kent Mental Health Services, Inc.

Versluys, H. (1980). The remediation of role disorders through focused group work. American Journal of Occupational Therapy 34(9): 609–614.

Webb, L. J. (1973). The therapeutic social club. American Journal of Occupational Therapy 27(2): 81–83.

Werner, V., Maddigan, R. F., and Watson, C. G. (1969). A study of two treatment programs for chronic mentally ill patients in occupational therapy. American Journal of Occupational Therapy 23(2): 132–136.

West, W. L. (ed.) (1959). Changing Concepts and Practices in Psychiatric Occupational Therapy. Dubuque, IA: William C. Brown.

White, C. V. (1953). Group projects with psychiatric patients. American Journal of Occupational Therapy 7(6): 253, 270.

Wiebe, R. H. (1967). The Search for Order 1877–1920. New York: Hill and Wang.

Wilson, L. G. (1979). The use of a stroke group treatment program on an extended care unit. The Canadian Journal of Occupational Therapy 46(1): 19–20.

Woodside, H. H. (1971). Occupational therapy—A historical perspective. The development of occupational therapy 1910–1929. American Journal of Occupational Therapy 25(5): 226–230.

Chapter **3**
Group Practice in the Wellness Era: 1900s–2000+

A comprehensive view of occupational therapy groups requires a broad historical perspective and an assessment of contemporary and emerging practice. The brief history in Chapter 2 described the stages through which group work in occupational therapy has evolved. In the development of any discipline or institution, one era builds on an earlier one so that the new exhibits characteristics of the earlier stages.

The early 1900s showed an increased number of occupational therapists working in the community rather than in medical facilities. Occupational therapy in the school systems, in a nonmedical environment, became the fastest growing branch of the profession. Gradually, in response to issues related to healthcare reform, managed care, and a shift of many important services from medical institutions to community programs, occupational therapists moved their service delivery into the community. This transition to community-based practice brought about a closer relationship between client and therapist. Dressler and MacRae (1998) wrote, "Therapists work with clients to develop skills, habits and volition necessary to gain power to make decisions and to take action in their own lives. More important, . . . clients set their own goals. Clients are seen as active agents and participants in their own treatment" (pp. 36–37).

The empowerment of clients to take an active role in healthcare, in the design and development of new programs and services, represents a new era in occupational therapy, which has been named the Wellness Era. Johnson (1986) defines the term 'wellness' as follows: "Wellness provides an opportunity for people to seek assistance with their problems of living and adapting and to create new options and solutions without acquiring a diagnostic label in the process of doing so. It also provides an opportunity for people who see themselves as whole complete individuals who, on occasion, have problems and who seek help in a supportive environment" (p. 13).

In the Wellness Era, the focus of group work has shifted from diagnosis or pathology to an emphasis on the health of the individual, on the inborn capacity for wholeness and well-being that exists in every person and can be supported and developed through the use of groups engaged in occupation. These groups must be versed in an understanding of group dynamics, an awareness of the importance of ego building, and a supportive context for therapeutic and educational change to occur.

With the rapidly changing pattern of the health delivery system (Box 3-1), corresponding changes have occurred in how occupational therapy services are provided. Occupational therapists are working in an expanding number of systems: educational systems, community-based social systems, medical systems, and even in the business arena. Although the goals of occupational therapy groups have not changed dramatically, the context and the locale where the groups are to be found, as well as the role of the occupational therapist and the population served, have expanded considerably. The following section will describe group work in the Wellness Era and present examples of currently evolving practice.

Group Practices

Given the changing conditions of healthcare delivery, what was the effect on occupational therapy group work? Was "occupation" still a major focus of occupational therapy group treatment? To answer these and other questions, Duncombe and Howe (1985 and 1995), researched the nature and scope of group work in the occupational therapy profession by surveying two random samples of practicing therapists in the United States. A three-part questionnaire

---

Box 3-1
Domino Effect

Change in the healthcare system gives rise to adaptation and adjustments to occupational therapy services and consequently in the nature and use of groups.

was used for both surveys with minor changes. Respondents were asked for information about the facility where they worked, whether or not they used groups as a method of treatment, and if not, the reason why (Figure 3-1). In the third part, respondents were requested to provide information on as many as four treatment groups they led and to complete a checklist of the characteristics and goals of the groups. A group was defined as "an aggregate of people who share a common purpose which can be attained only by group members interacting and working together" (Mosey, 1973, p. 45).

Results from the first survey (120 respondents) provided information from 72 therapists who led groups and who reported on the 209 groups that they led. In the second survey (188 respondents), 92 therapists who led groups reported leading 233 different groups.

The descriptions of the groups fell into six major categories; however, there were clearly some areas of overlap in the activities used (Box 3-2). Overlapping is characteristic of the flexibility required in practice. The main types of groups were clustered as follows: four types of task groups, two types of discussion groups, exercise groups, self-expression groups, sensorimotor or sensory integration groups, and educational groups. Duncombe and Howe (1985) developed brief descriptions of 10 types of groups.

Types of Task Groups

Cooking Group
Cooking groups usually combined the tasks of planning, shopping, cooking, and eating a meal. These groups, having five to eight members, often cooked a meal for a much larger group. A majority of the cooking groups were therapy programs for adult and adolescent mental health patients. Cooking groups were also found in rehabilitation programs for persons with spinal cord injuries, arthritis, and neurological conditions.

These short-term, open or closed groups, had the specific goals of facilitating communication and socialization, increasing task skills, sharing information, and educating members.

Activities of Daily Living Group
This category contained the largest number of reported groups. Living skills groups were conducted in hospitals, clinics, daycare programs, nursing homes, and rehabilitation programs for adults with psychosocial dysfunctions, head and neurological injuries, stroke, and cardiovascular conditions. Depending on the settings, these groups shared two distinct sets of goals. Some groups worked on developing living skills or greater independence in self-care within the institution, whereas other groups worked on pre-discharge living skills and on preparation for independent living in the community. The daily living skills groups were predominantly closed, short-term groups with three to eight members and with specific goals to increase task skills and share information.

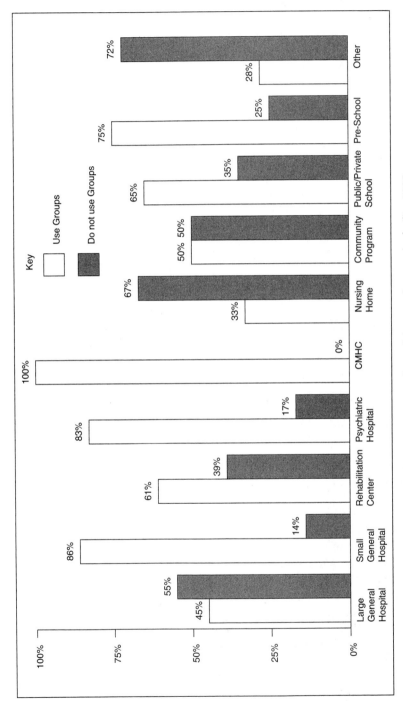

Figure 3-1. Percentage comparison of the use of groups by facility, 1995.

> ### Box 3-2
> ### Typing Groups
>
> The authors of the survey established 10 categories of groups that fell within six types:
>
> - the exercise group
> - task groups
> - the self-expression group
> - discussion groups
> - the sensorimotor or sensory integration group
> - the educational group

Arts and Crafts Group

Arts and crafts groups were typically used for the evaluation and treatment of psychosocial disorders. Members worked on individual projects within a group setting. Some of these groups—particularly those concerned with evaluation of existing skills—were small, with less than five members. Other groups, concerned with developing leisure skills, had as many as 15 members and were designed to increase task skills and promote socialization and communication between members.

Special Task Group

These task groups met to create a product other than a meal. They were used most often in community mental health and developmental disabilities programs for adults, as well as in after-school programs for children and adolescents. One type of task group worked on projects such as publishing a newsletter or a yearbook or planning and holding a recreational or social event. Another type of task group concentrated on prevocational or work-related assembly and production projects. Some task groups were small; others as large as 20 members. They were usually long-term, closed groups whose goals were to increase socialization and communication as well as task skills.

Self-Expression Group

The self-expression group was reported by therapists working with adults with psychosocial problems. The specific goals were for socialization and communication in small groups of fewer than 10 members. This group primarily used art modalities to encourage self-expression. At the time the second survey was completed, these groups mostly had been discontinued owing to changes in psychiatric treatment methods and to the criteria for reimbursement.

Exercise Group

Members of exercise groups were involved in doing physical exercise to increase coordination, mobility, and strength. Group activities consisted of games involving ball play such as catch, ping-pong, volleyball, and bowling. Also included were recreational sports and movement activities. Members often participated in these activities from a chair or a wheelchair. Group size varied from 6 to as many as 20, and participants were often adults with psychosocial, physical, or developmental disabilities. The primary goals for exercise groups were to increase physical abilities and to facilitate communication and socialization.

Discussion Group

Feeling-Oriented Discussion Group

These groups were usually found in mental health programs and were sometimes designated as group psychotherapy. Role-playing, poetry, and fantasy often promoted discussion. Activities included such modalities as self-awareness and self-esteem work, grief work, and anger management. The goals of the discussion groups were to provide support, increase communication and socialization, and achieve insight. These groups were small verbal groups of 6 to 10 adults.

Reality-Oriented Discussion Group

The reality-oriented discussion group was designed for adults and the elderly. Topics for discussion included current events, the daily news, events concerning the program, individual treatment goals, the use of time, and program or discharge planning. Some groups used specific group techniques such as assertiveness training and role-playing. Groups were predominantly verbal, short-term, and open or closed, and the goals were to increase communication and socialization, provide education, and share information.

Sensorimotor and Sensory Integration Group

These groups were for preschool through high-school children who were receiving group treatment in school or after-school programs. Problems ranged from learning disabilities, cerebral palsy, developmental disorders, auditory problems, and/or visual problems. Group members participated in gross and fine motor activities, as well as in touch, taste, and movement activities. Groups were predominantly long-term and the goals were to develop physical abilities, improve sensory integration, and provide opportunities for communication and socialization.

Educational Group

The majority of the educational groups were for parents and families of individuals receiving treatment. Also included were groups that provided information and discussion on medications, joint protection for arthritis, and family effectiveness. These were verbal, short-term groups with goals to provide support and meet health needs, to teach, and to share information.

> •• **Sidebar 3-1**
> *Definitions*
>
> **Task skills:** *Skills needed to complete a given act, job, or performance*
>
> **Reality-Oriented Group:** *A group whose goal is to identify and discuss issues that are occurring in the current lives of its members*
>
> **Feeling-Oriented Group:** *A group whose goal is to promote and discuss the feelings of its members*
>
> **Socialization:** *To promote behavior that encourages social interaction*

Discussion of Survey Results

During the 10-year period between the time when the first and second surveys were completed, the types of groups led by occupational therapists showed little change except for a decrease in the number of mental health groups such as the self-expression group and the feeling-oriented discussion groups. In part, this was a result of the medical changes in the treatment of psychiatric conditions and the changes in the reimbursement guidelines for those types of groups.

A trend showed an increase in occupational therapists employed in school programs and in programs labeled "other." These "other" programs included community programs such as home treatment, private practice, outpatient clinics, and early intervention. Concurrently, there was a decrease in the number of therapists working in psychiatric hospitals. This trend paralleled the demographic changes in the profession (American Occupational Therapy Association, 1991; Price, 1993), and reflected a trend away from primarily medical-based practice to a community-based practice. This is of particular interest because it raises the potential for the development of new areas of practice such as groups designed to promote health and wellness for people of all ages (Strickland, 1991).

Although some things changed during the 10-year period between the first and second survey, others remained the same. Occupational therapy groups continued to be small groups of 6 to 10 members rather than larger groups and continued to include a significantly greater number of activity groups than verbal groups. Both of these findings were statistically significant ($P<.01$) (Box 3-3).

The most commonly listed group goal was to increase performance skills, namely task skills, cognitive skills, and physical skills. Although the therapists identified the types of groups that they were leading, often no clear difference existed between categories regarding naming group activities. The identical activities were used for achieving different goals. For instance, both the exercise groups and the sensorimotor/sensory integration groups included similar activities such as exercises, games, and gross and fine motor activities to increase strength, balance, sensory processing, and dexterity. However, sensory inte-

Box 3-3
OT Group Characteristics

Small group size: 4 to 6 members

Types: More activity groups than verbal groups

Group goals: To facilitate communication and socialization and increase task skills and physical abilities

gration groups also incorporated traditional sensory integration treatment approaches, such as vestibular, tactile, and proprioceptive stimulation, into group activities.

Overlapping activities were used in cooking groups, daily living groups, and task groups. The activities of these groups were similar but with different purposes/meaning to clients or context. For example, cooking may be seen as a life skill task, a leisure interest or hobby, an emotionally meaningful task, or as a task used to develop work skills. Activities in the task groups were more leisure and vocationally oriented, whereas the activities of daily living groups were more self-care oriented; however, all were directed at increasing skills for independent living in the present milieu, be it in a group facility or an independent living arrangement in the community.

The therapists responding to the survey indicated that facilitating communication and socialization were some of the most important goals for their groups. In discussing concepts from socialization theory, Burke (1983) stated, "Socialization offers the useful perspective that persons acquire behavior in the process of being exposed to role models, expectations, demands for performance, and information about performance. Socialization aids development of a new and appropriate thinking and behaving throughout the life span. . . . " (p. 136). Clearly, communication is an essential component of group participation, and increased communication contributes to greater learning in the group experience. Socialization also involves the interactional process between individuals and alleviates isolation. In the Wellness Era, socialization plays an important part in assisting individuals to adjust to new circumstances and to achieve and maintain health. Whether the group is for the treatment of physical or emotional problems, or both, the emphasis continues to be on increasing skills through structured learning experiences as it had been in the prior decades (Box 3-4).

Occupational therapy is not alone in stressing the value of small support groups in promoting wellness and successful living in the community. The field of medicine has recently published many studies showing that the incidence of both recovery from illness and prevention of illness were higher among individuals who were involved in socialization and support groups (Ornish, 1999). Ornish said, "Group support may be particularly beneficial in cancer patients.

> **Box 3-4**
> **Activity Qualities**
>
> These two surveys indicate that most occupational therapy groups focus on activities that increase occupational skills and adaptation. While one activity can be used for achieving different goals, the following are some of the qualities of the activity that need to be considered before using it as a group activity:
>
> - The skill level of the clients in areas of physical, cognitive, and social-emotional functioning
> - The group's interest in this activity
> - The physical setting where the group meets
> - Environmental constraints related to space, noise, time, equipment, etc.
> - Activity constraints related to age, culture, language, and educational level
> - The goals of this activity and whether they conflict with other group goals
> - Other important considerations

People who have been recently diagnosed with cancer may find it hard to get emotional support when they most need it" (p. 57). A similar statement was made by Dossey (1999): "Social contact was proved to be an important factor in resisting all major diseases" (p. 165).

Reimbursement Issues

The final section of the questionnaire (Duncombe and Howe, 1995) provided data on reimbursement and documentation of group treatment. The question of documentation practices showed that 94% of the respondents maintained individual documentation for patients receiving group treatment, whereas only five respondents indicated keeping documentation on both the individuals and the group. Although documentation of the group process may not be important for reimbursement, it becomes important as a record of the efficacy of occupational therapy group treatment. Therefore, the need to develop proper documentation procedures for the group's process as a database for the justification of group treatment as a modality is of critical importance. Occupational therapists need to know how to focus treatment on functional outcomes and how to measure changes in behavior. Chapter 5 presents several methods for evaluating group processes.

Almost one half of the same respondents stated that they charged clients the same fee for individual as for group treatment, thus making group treatment a more cost-effective treatment. Trahey (1991) actually documented a one-third decrease in labor costs by using group treatment rather than individual treatment with patients receiving hip replacement therapy. Given the economic advantages that accrue from group treatment and the pressures in occupational therapy departments to handle more patients with less staff, it is likely that group treatment will continue to flourish as it did in the recession years of the 1970s and in the depression years of the 1930s and 1940s. Trahey (1991) admonished, "We must not allow the pressures of cost containment and personnel shortages to compromise our efforts to provide quality care and promote the quality of life of our patients" (p. 400). In her study, Trahey (1991) also emphasized that her group was led by an experienced, well-trained occupational therapist. A less-trained staff person carrying out this job, even under the supervision of a highly competent therapist, may not achieve the same results.

The history of occupational therapy groups presented in Chapter 2 frequently refers to the impact that economic factors have on group treatment practices. The period from the late 1980s to the present time has been a time of fiscal retrenchment and cost containment. Healthcare costs have been paid by government, state, and local funding; by third-party payers, usually insurance groups; and by healthcareconsumers. To compete for healthcare dollars, occupational therapy needs to prove the efficacy of its services and to show functional improvements in clients by quantifying progress using concrete outcomes whenever possible. The pressure to document outcomes of treatment is likely only to increase under current healthcare plans. A distinction needs to be made here between types of practice in which real, interacting groups are deliberately used by a therapist, and the simultaneous model of service delivery. Under the pressure for increased productivity, therapists may treat several patients simultaneously, seating them apart from each other and moving from one to another, but without planning activities that elicit cooperative work toward a common goal, or even encouraging verbal interaction among patients. This is often called "group treatment," but is actually one-on-one treatment.

Evolving Practice in the Wellness Era

The healthcare system in the United States continues to change both for the patients seeking care and for the professionals providing that care. Occupational therapy services are undergoing changes as well. Streib (1999) published the results of a survey of occupational therapy practitioners detailing their employment situations. This study was taken from a self-selected sample of 100 registered occupational therapists and occupational therapy assistants who were asked where they currently worked. Many of the respondents indicated that they worked in primarily medical settings such as hospitals, nursing facilities, outpatient treatment, or home health. Others were working for school systems in the community. However, approximately 40% of the respondents checked "other."

This study showed a continuing trend toward a greater number of occupational therapy practitioners working in community-based, nonmedical settings.

Examples of group work conducted by occupational therapists in community-based practice include preschool and school-based programs for children, programming for the elderly, groups with juveniles, family work, community vocational services, and support groups. Support groups may have occupational therapists as leaders, or they may be member-led with occupational therapists working in consulting or teaching roles.

The limited number of programs in which students can gain experience working with client groups has led faculty members to organize and supervise occupational therapy groups in areas of community service previously not familiar with occupational therapy. One such program was developed by Scott (1999) who states the following: "Sites included a shelter for women who were homeless and mentally ill, senior programs for well-elderly persons and persons with mental illness, an in-patient pediatric sickle-cell unit and a university health club with programs for students and staff members" (p. 569). In a smoking cessation program, the students co-led support groups to "help members cope with the pressures of nicotine withdrawal and lifestyle changes supplemented with deep breathing techniques and relaxation tapes supplied by the American Lung Association" (Scott, 1999, p. 570).

Anecdotal evidence showed that during the late 1990s and into the millenium, major changes occurred in service delivery. The examples that follow are evidence of shifts toward community-based occupational therapy.

In many communities, there are programs for the elderly to help them maintain wellness, sustain their level of function, and prevent social deprivation. In such programs, occupational therapists organize small activity groups that can combine socialization with the functional and recreational skills that help to maintain the individual's self-esteem. These programs often include an educational component concerning nutrition, exercise, and community resources. For example, occupational therapy was included as part of a well-elderly program organized in a Los Angeles area for residents of subsidized apartment complexes for residents 60 years or older living independently. In addition to a 2-hour weekly group session, each participant engaged in an hour per month one-on-one interaction with the therapist "for developing customized plans for lifestyle redesign in which the participants were encouraged to creatively employ occupation in a personalized way to adapt to the challenges associated with aging" (1998, Jackson et al., p. 327). The participants joined in a four-part group process consisting of didactic presentations, peer exchanges, direct experience, and personal exploration. The elders who joined this program exhibited gains in physical health, physical functioning, social functioning, vitality, mental health, and life satisfaction.

In South Carolina, an occupational therapist answered an advertisement that called for someone with a background in human services to be coordinator of resident services in an apartment complex for low-income persons older than 55 years. She found that her responsibilities were threefold:

- To help residents meet any individual need, such as transportation;
- To promote a sense of community in the complex; Womack and Farmer (1999) stated, "This takes the form of providing group opportunities for residents to engage in meaningful occupations, varying the physical environment, and encouraging awareness of neighbors' strengths and needs" (p. 19); and
- To develop a program for residents in which she brought in resource persons from the community to provide information and support.

Although this position did not call specifically for an occupational therapist's knowledge and skills, in reality it contained the essence of occupational therapy practice. With the expansion of occupational therapists working in community programs, many therapists will be working where their knowledge and skills, not their titles, are valued.

Occupational therapy training provides the ideal combination of task management and group process skills in a community mental health program in the San Francisco area. The therapist was assigned the task of working with a pre-employment cooking group of members that cooked lunch once a week for all the program members. She also helped this group start a catering service. Her knowledge of group process and task analysis made her especially valuable to the program. In the past, the individuals hired in her position were either cooking specialists who did not know how to work with a group or persons who were proficient in group process but could not organize the cooking tasks.

One community agency in the Southwest introduced occupational therapy to answer the extensive mental health needs of young people incarcerated in a juvenile detention center. Presented problems included learning disorders, hyperactivity, affective disorders, anxiety, and substance abuse. Unfortunately, most staff members of correctional institutions were not trained in adolescent development, task analysis, or group process. Youths under detention benefit from participating in planned group activities as a means of learning more adaptive coping skills and socially appropriate methods of peer interaction. In addition, groups help with understanding the expectations of the correctional system. Occupational therapists' skills in observation and evaluation can provide information regarding individuals' specific skills deficiencies and areas requiring special attention (Abras, 1999).

Another program for young people is the University of Southern California youth program, which is based on principles of occupation. The program examines how gang behavior or membership relates to identity and even survival. The occupational therapists are effective at addressing what is meaningful for these youths and what has purpose for individuals and groups.

Work with family or community living groups is being emphasized in current practice. Families occupy an important role in the lives of individuals with disabilities, and therapists need to be more aware of this focus (Humphry, Gonzales, and Taylor, 1993). Family and parent groups have long been a part of occupational therapy with infants and children, and now this participation has been extended to the care of aging parents. Frequently the family needs to be brought as a group to address the care and support needed by aging parents or relatives. An arrangement that is agreeable to all concerned often needs to be worked out. A care arrangement may involve developing a plan whereby family members can share the care of the relative. Sometimes the plan may require moving the relative to an environment that provides more extensive services. When there are serious health problems, several meetings may be required before a satisfactory arrangement may be worked out. The occupational therapist's role in this process is to coordinate and lead the group as well as one who can contribute and interpret information to the group.

Community centers frequently sponsor groups for individuals who have been discharged from treatment programs but still desire or need group support. There are support groups addressing mental health concerns; specific health-related problems such as diabetes, AIDS, and cancer; and post–addiction treatment concerns. Some of these groups are organized as leaderless groups; in these, the occupational therapist assumes the role of an organizing guide or contributing member. In other groups, the role may vary from facilitator to group leader.

An example of a peer-developed support group is a group in the Boston area for persons with head injuries. The 13 members have been meeting every 2 weeks for 16 months. It is an open group. A participant observer in this group, Schwartzberg writes

> Many of the positive attributes of the group seem similar to processes found in successful peer support groups. These attributes include believing and feeling part of the group because members have a common problem and can validate the effects of the injury by sharing and receiving information in a variety of ways through the group. (1994, p. 279)

Just as many other peer support groups, this group is self-governing and self-regulating, and its members share a common condition, situation, symptoms, and experiences. "Knowledge of the functional aspects of disability, community resources, and group activity analysis and adaptation techniques enable occupational therapists to easily assume unique roles in support groups for persons with head injury in helping to establish, facilitate, or act as advocates with such groups" (Schwartzberg, 1994, p. 304).

The recent enactment of welfare reform with its emphasis on economic independence through employment in the private sector, presents new and challenging openings for occupational therapists. Kathy Parker, OTR (1999) states that "OTs are well-equipped to coach clients in skills needed for employment—everything from managing time to practicing good social skills. They can also advise employers on how to accommodate persons with cultural, social, or learning impairments" (p. 8). Despite the opportunities for the expertise of occupational therapy in this area, to date few occupational therapists are working there (Parker, 1999).

In the community programs described above, the occupational therapist has had to learn to work without the traditional supports available in medical facilities, and to move into areas of health and wellness. A crucial element of

Box 3-5
Community Partnerships

Community-based occupational therapists must form partnerships with others who have vested interests in supporting the clients.

this type of group work is developing "an entrepreneurial perspective by acquiring skills that have currency in the marketplace not limited by medical necessity" (Fine, 1998, p.14). Community programs have seldom included an occupational therapist in their staffing pattern; hence, special funds often need to be obtained to employ them (Box 3-5). The occupational therapist must be free of old organizational dependencies and able to clearly articulate the knowledge, goals, and skills of occupational therapy services. These need to be marketed specifically to the particular needs of the clients and agency, and should include data from research or outcome studies of the success of similar types of group work in occupational therapy programs.

The variety of programs in the community where occupational therapy groups enrich the health and quality of life of individual continues to broaden. This in no way implies that we should abandon what has traditionally been successful in medical and rehabilitation programs. Rather, the profession needs to broaden its scope, its vision, and areas of practice. As Fidler stated," As a profession, our single focus on an identity as a therapy, as a remedial rehabilitation service, has, I believe, significantly hampered our development. This narrow identity has, over many years, hindered our discovery and validation of the rich and broad dimensions of occupation" (Fidler, 2000, p. 99).

Conclusion

In this chapter, two surveys of occupational therapy practice have been presented to give a perspective of practice in the Wellness Era. Examples of community-based occupational therapy practice that reflect the growing edge of the profession augment this picture. The field of occupational therapy is striving to document the efficacy of its services, and the area of group treatment is no exception. Documentation should emphasize that occupational therapy group treatment is making an occupational, as well as a qualitative, difference in the client's life.

Review Questions

1. The two surveys of occupational therapy group practice showed that there were significantly more activity groups than verbal groups. What other distinguishing features of occupational therapy groups were found regarding group size? Group goals?

2. Have the changes in healthcare and reimbursement of the past 10 years influenced the practice of occupational therapy? From the trends stated in these studies, what are some of the changes occurring in occupational therapy group treatment?
3. What are the types of patients involved in group treatment?
4. Where is the location of treatment?
5. What are the goals of group treatment?
6. What is the cost of group treatment?
7. What are the methods of payment for group treatment?
8. How has the role of the group activity changed in the Wellness Era?
9. What types of groups have been used in the Wellness Era?
10. Why have certain types of groups been used more than other types?
11. What questions would you pose to demonstrate the effectiveness of occupational groups in the Wellness Era?

References

Abras, T. (1999) Meeting mental health needs of adolescents. OT Week, 13(18): 8–9.

American Occupational Therapy Association (1991). Member Data Survey—1990 (1991). Rockville, MD: American Occupational Therapy Association.

Burke, J. P. (1983). Defining occupation: Importing and organizing interdisciplinary knowledge. In G. Kielhofner (ed.), Health Through Occupation: Theory and Practice in Occupational Therapy. Philadelphia: F. A. Davis.

Dossey, L. (1999). Reinventing Medicine. New York: Harper Collins.

Dressler, J. & MacRae, A. (1998). Advocacy, partnership and client-centered practice in California. Occupational Therapy in Mental Health 14 (1/2). New York: The Haworth Press.

Duncombe, L., and Howe, M. C. (1985). Group work in occupational therapy: A survey of practice. American Journal of Occupational Therapy 39(3): 163–170.

Duncombe, L., and Howe, M. C. (1995). Group treatment: Goals, tasks, and economic implications. American Journal of Occupational Therapy, 49: 199–205.

Fidler, G. (2000). Beyond the therapy model—building a future. American Journal of Occupational Therapy 54(1): 99–101.

Fine, S. B. (1998). Surviving the health care revolution: Rediscovering the meaning of "Good Work." In Occupational Therapy in Mental Health, 14(1/2): 14.

Humphry, R., Gonzalez, S., and Taylor, E. (1993). Family involvement in practice: Issues and attitudes. American Journal of Occupational Therapy 47: 587–593.

Jackson, J., Carlson, M., Mandel, D., Zemke, R., Clark, F. (1998). Occupation in lifestyle redesign: The well elderly study occupational therapy study program. American Journal of Occupational Therapy, 25(5): 326–336.

Johnson, J. A. (1986). Wellness: A context for living. Thorofare, N.J.: Slack Inc.

Mosey, A. C. (1973). Activities Therapy. New York: Raven Press.

Ornish, D. (1998). Love and Survival. New York: Harper Collins.

Parker, K. (1999). In Johansson, C. Getting America up and working. OT Week, 13(14): 8–11.

Price, S. (1993). The issue is new pathways for psychosocial occupational therapy. American Journal of Occupational Therapy 47: 557–560.

Schwartzberg, S. (1994). Helping factors in a peer-developed support group for persons with head injury. American Journal of Occupational Therapy, 48(4): 297–304.

Scott, A. H. (1999). Wellness works: Community service health promotion groups led by occupational therapy students. American Journal of Occupational Therapy, 53(6): 566–574.

Streib, P. (1999). Survey: Most practitioners holding their own. OT Week, 13(10): 8–10.

Strickland, R. (1991) Nationally speaking: Directions for the future—Occupational therapy practice then and now, 1949–the present. American Journal of Occupational Therapy, 45: 105–107.

Trahey, P. J. (1991). A comparison of the cost-effectiveness of two types of occupational therapy services. American Journal of Occupational Therapy 45: 397–401.

Womack, J. & Farmer, P. (1999). Strong roots, flexible branches. OT Practice, 4(10): 17–21.

Chapter **4**
A Model for Group Work

In the preceding chapters, we described many different kinds of groups and examined their characteristics and overall goals. This chapter describes a model for an occupational therapy group; the model is titled "the functional group" (Box 4-1). The model was first introduced in the 1986 edition of this book. It is being presented here in greater detail that reflects the model's evolution and refinement since its inception.

The functional group model is presented in accordance with a framework established by Reed (1984). In her description of the process of developing practice models, Reed identifies eight elements fundamental to the process:

1. the frame of reference
2. assumptions
3. concepts
4. expected results of intervention

Box 4-1
The Functional Group

The functional group, based on a functional approach to group work, is empirically derived from clinical experience and research.

---

5. assessment instruments
6. intervention strategies
7. logical deductions
8. intervention principles

Just as any research process, the functional group model is incomplete in a strict sense. Although based on empirical data, the model has not been completely tested; therefore, we lack total evidence for the final element: intervention principles. Nevertheless, the model functions to organize occupational therapy group practice, education, and research. Applications and research evidence pointing to the accuracy of the model will be summarized in Chapter 10.

Framework of the Model

Frame of Reference

The functional group model is based on research in five areas (Box 4-2) related to occupational therapy:

1. group dynamics
2. effectance
3. needs hierarchy
4. purposeful activity
5. adaptation

Group dynamics—the domain of social scientists—concerns the interrelationships of persons in a small group. The belief that a psychological field, just as an energy field, acts on and affects the behavior of a group was raised by Kurt Lewin in the 1930s (Knowles and Knowles, 1972). "Effectance" refers to the belief that individuals are drawn toward activity and that this behavior is self-motivated. The term "needs hierarchy" refers to the belief that humans have many needs and these are arranged in order of importance. Purposeful activity

Box 4-2
Base in Research

Research in the following areas related to occupational therapy forms the basis for the functional group model:

- group dynamics
- effectance
- needs hierarchy
- purposeful activity
- adaptation

has come to be recognized as closely related to satisfaction of needs, and adaptation is recognized as one goal of this activity. Let us examine more closely each of these five areas.

Much of the early literature on group dynamics was important to developing the functional group model. By understanding the normal group, we formulated ideas about the therapy group and then the functional group. Concepts central to the beliefs regarding group dynamics were derived from Bales' (1950) work on interaction analysis and Benne and Sheats' (1978) description of group membership and leadership functions. Additional works on group dynamics, such as those on group cohesiveness (Cartwright and Zander, 1968; Yalom, 1970), the phases of group development (Bennis and Shepard, 1956; Garland, Jones, and Kolodny, 1965; Tuckman, 1965), and individual growth through group process (Lifton, 1961), were also used to develop the model.

If we understand how persons within groups interact, we can increase the benefits of group participation for individuals (Box 4-3). We should keep in mind several basic principles of group dynamics:

- Groups have a common goal and dynamic interaction between members. Through use of the information base available in a group, members are provided with a here-and-now reality orientation that encourages growth and change. Groups can enhance the use of occupations to help people function independently, that is, to adapt to the environment or adapt the environment to them.
- Groups provide multiple feedback and support. Groups are designed to give the amount and type of feedback and support that members need. Feedback and support are part of the process of doing and participating in the group activities selected to meet individual and social needs.
- Groups promote independence from and decreased dependence on an externally designated leader in a developmental progression. Group discussions and activities can be structured to encourage group-centered leadership. Structuring activities and the environment so that nonhuman objects lead the action gives members an opportunity to learn about what the environment can do and their own capabilities.
- Groups support growth and change of members. Through discussion and participation in growth activities, groups can encourage and promote growth and change of members. By selecting activities that permit practice and learning of skills needed to achieve mastery and competency, groups can provide opportunities for growth and change of members.
- Groups have a capacity for self-direction. Groups can be organized to accommodate many levels of human development and functioning. Enabling the group to lead the doing by giving members a set of possibilities empowers the group's capacity for self-direction.
- Groups can satisfy individual needs and social demands. Through discussion and activities, groups can satisfy individual needs and provide learning necessary for the fulfillment of social demands. Groups can be used to

Box 4-3
Functional Group Correlates

Group dynamics is governed by basic principles, among them that groups:

- have a common goal and dynamic interaction between members,
- provide multiple feedback and support,
- promote independence from and decreased dependence on the leader,
- support growth and change of members,
- have a capacity for self-direction, and
- can satisfy individual needs and social demands.

Among the principles applying to the more specific therapy group are that groups:

- provide a here-and-now, reality orientation that encourages growth and change,
- are designed to give the amount and type of feedback and support that members need,
- can be structured to encourage group-centered leadership,
- can lead to individual growth and change,
- can be organized to accommodate many levels of human development and functioning, and
- can satisfy individual needs and provide learning necessary to fulfill social demands.

The occupation-specific functional group is influenced by the following principles, that:

- groups can enhance the use of occupations to help people function independently by adapting to the environment or adapting the environment to them
- feedback and support are part of the process of doing and participating
- structuring activities and the environment so that nonhuman objects lead the action permits members to learn about the environment and their own capabilities
- selection of activities that permit practice and learning of skills needed to achieve mastery and competency, can lead to growth and change in members
- enabling the group to lead the doing by giving members a set of possibilities, empowers the group's capacity for self-direction, and
- groups can be used to maintain, improve, or enhance the occupational nature of people by providing members the opportunity to deal with the real functions of objects.

maintain, improve, or enhance the occupational nature of people by providing members an opportunity to deal with the real functions of objects.

Robert White's (1959, 1971) work on "effectance motivation" or the "urge toward competence" was also central to the development of our model. Simply stated, White believed that exploratory behavior was self-motivated; he coined the term effectance to describe this motivation. This behavior had "adaptive value," White (1959) said. "Effectance motivation must be conceived to involve satisfaction—a feeling of efficacy—in transactions in which behavior has an exploratory, varying, experimental character. . . . The behavior leads the organism to find out how the environment can be changed and what consequences flow from these changes" (p. 329). Maslow (1970) also attempted to explain motivation. According to him, humans have "intrinsic growth tendencies."

Maslow stated that people have "basic needs" that are organized in a hierarchy. These basic needs are as follows:

- physiological
- safety
- belongingness and love
- esteem
- self-actualization

In Maslow's view, unsatisfied needs are a source of motivation; the individual puts his or her energies into satisfying needs, dealing with the various needs in the order given.

Mosey (1973) similarly described a needs hierarchy in her concept of "health needs." She noted, "health needs are defined as inherent human requirements that must be met in order for an individual to experience a sense of physical, psychological, and social well-being" (p. 14). In Mosey's terminology, these needs are psycho-physical, security, love and acceptance, group association, esteem, sexual, developmental, and pleasure (pp. 14–15). Mosey believes that a "need-satisfying environment" is an essential backdrop to a treatment program oriented toward change (Box 4-4).

An idea central to the functional group model is purposeful activity. King (1978) defines purposeful activities as those that encourage an "adaptive response." In Reed's (1984) view, purposeful activities, or "meaningful occupations," give direction to "goal-oriented" behavior. Although Reed acknowl-

---

Box 4-4
O.T. Role

Because patients are often unable to meet their own health needs, the occupational therapist must engineer need-satisfying environments in conjunction with change-oriented programs.

edges that the definition of a term such as meaningful is usually subjective, she states that "among the possible needs or demands which activities could fulfill are physiologic, security, belonging, societal and self-actualizing needs" (p. 502). Regardless of the needs they fulfill, according to Reed, all purposeful activities have an intent and are practical in daily living.

In his studies regarding intrinsic rewards and motivation, Csikszentmihalyi (1975, 1990), gives further insight into the purpose or value of activity. He believes that people experience a "flow state" when their "skills match with the opportunities for action in the environment" (p. 177). When there is a mismatch, stress, worry, or boredom may result. The flow state also increases the individual's feelings of being in control of his/her actions. On such occasions the individual feels a great sense of enjoyment. Csikszentmihalyi (1990) calls this an "optimal experience" (p. 3). He describes an optimal experience as: "a sense that one's skills are adequate to cope with the challenges at hand, in a goal-directed, rule-bound, action system that provides clear clues as to how well one is performing. Concentration is so intense that there is no attention left to think about anything irrelevant, or to worry about problems" (p. 71). This theory about flow has generated ideas for the design of activities in some occupational therapy programs (Box 4-5).

Fidler and Fidler (1978) explain purposeful action in their concept of "doing." "Doing is viewed as enabling the development and integration of the sensory, motor, cognitive, and psychological systems; serving as a socializing agent, and verifying one's efficacy as a competent, contributing member of one's society" (p. 305). They also emphasize that "both the quality and variety of doing is critical for ego development and adaptation" (p. 308). Barris, Kielhofner, and Hawkins (1983) also point out that intrinsically motivated behaviors lead to feelings of personal satisfaction.

Finally, to varying degrees all of the literature cited above touches on human adaptation. According to Burke (1983), "occupation [is] . . . a behavior which is motivated by an intrinsic, conscious urge to be effective in the environment in order to enact a variety of individually interpreted roles that are shaped by cultural tradition and learned through the process of socialization" (p. 136). For Reed (1984), "adaptation through occupation . . . means the or-

Box 4-5
Integrating Flow

"Flow helps to integrate the self because in that state of deep concentration consciousness is usually well ordered. Thoughts, intentions, feelings and all the senses are focused on the same goal. Experience is in harmony. And when the flow episode is over, one feels more "together" than before, not only internally but also with respect to other people and to the world in general" (p. 41).

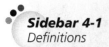

Sidebar 4-1
Definitions

Adaptation: *Any changes in the structure, habits, or behavior of individuals that lead to their adjustment to their environment*

Adaptive response: *The process by which persons adjust to the demands of their environment*

ganization and management of occupational activities and tasks in a manner that meets the goal of achieving maximum autonomy or functional independence, actualization or satisfaction and accomplishment" (p. 495). King (1978) and Fidler and Fidler (1978) see purposeful activity, or "doing," as primary to adaptation. White (1959) surmises that "effectance motivation" has adaptive value, and Maslow (1970) considers "basic needs" as intrinsic to the organization of adaptive human behavior: physiological, psychological, and social.

As stated previously, the frame of reference for the functional group model includes research findings on group dynamics, effectance, needs hierarchy, purposeful activity, and adaptation. In addition, a significant relationship exists between these beliefs (K. L. Reed, personal communication, July 22, 1984). The model assumes a relationship between groups, therapy, and occupation. By examining the normal (nonspecific) group, we can better grasp variations in the therapy (more specific) group and then apply the concepts to the functional (occupation-specific) group.

Assumptions

Assumptions are ideas we accept as valid or true without having proof or logical support. Each of us accepts certain assumptions whether or not we are aware of doing so. Again following Reed's (1984) framework for model development, we describe the assumptions in forming the functional group model. The assumptions are organized into four groups:

- humans (Box 4-6)
- health (Box 4-7)
- occupation (Box 4-8)
- therapy (Box 4-9)

Concepts

At the heart of the model is a set of concepts that define the model in precise terms. The basic concepts here are adaptation and occupation (or action) and its four different forms: purposeful action, self-initiated action, spontaneous or here-and-now action, and group-centered action.

Box 4-6
People Assumptions

In this model we make nine assumptions about people. That:

- People are bio-psycho-social systems.
- People are social beings and therefore exist in groups.
- People are action or "doing" oriented, motivated toward competency.
- People have needs that can be met through the give and take of a social system such as a group.
- People communicate socially (interact) both verbally and nonverbally.
- Growth and change are processes inherent in life.
- People are unique, complete individuals, with wholeness or congruence between emotion and action.
- Groups exist as models of the social behavior patterns in the larger society.
- Groups mobilize powerful forces that have important effects on people as individuals: Senses of identity are shaped by groups; positions in the group affect safety and self-esteem; and group membership may be highly valued or seen as a burden to the individual.

The functional group is defined by the use of time and energy in action designed to promote adaptation. Adaptation is defined as the adjustment of the organism to its environment or the process by which it adjusts (Reed and Sanderson, 1983). Fitness and health are terms used to describe a state of adaptation. The characteristics of adaptation (King, 1978) have been translated into the functional group model shown in Table 4-1.

Box 4-7
Health Assumptions

In this model, we make four assumptions about health. That:

- An individual's state of health involves mind, body (internal), and physical environment—the individual in interaction with the social and physical environment.
- Purposeful activity supports the health of mind and body in an individual and a collective being.
- Health involves a state of independence and capacity for self-direction.
- Health involves a state of interdependence and capacity for relatedness.

Box 4-8
Occupations Assumptions

In this model, we make six assumptions about occupation. That:

- Directed purposeful occupations used in a group experience encourage the person to assume responsibility for meeting individual needs.
- Purposeful activities involve choice or volition by the individual and group toward a goal or purpose.
- Purposeful activities, or occupations, used in a group experience are useful in improving the performance level and adaptive behavior of the person and thus increasing potential for meeting individual responsibilities.
- Active doing (involvement) in a group encourages the maintenance, development, and redevelopment of skills in areas of self-care, productivity (work), and leisure (play).
- Through active doing in a group experience, the individual gains a sense of self-worth and self-appraisal.
- Lack of purposeful activity or idleness in a group leads to disorientation and breakdown in habits and thus threatens the individual health of both mind and body.

Box 4-9
Therapy Assumptions

We make three assumptions about therapy. That:

- Occupational therapy conducted in a group involves the use of directed, purposeful occupations or activities to positively influence a person's sense of well-being or state of health.
- Occupational therapy conducted in a group elicits an adaptive response and thereby requires a positive role that involves active participation; requires the person to meet the environmental demands of needs, tasks, and goals; permits subcortical centers to integrate and organize a response; leads to self-reinforcement (King, 1978).
- Occupational therapy conducted in a group attempts to satisfy individual biological, psychological, and social requirements in conjunction with efforts to influence change in the person's state of health.

Table 4-1
Adaptation and the Functional Group Model

Characteristics of Adaptation*	Functional Group Model
Requires a role that involves active participation	Group empowers maximum involvement through inter-action between members, a common goal, and a task.
	Group mobilizes powerful forces that have important effects on member's sense of individual and group identity.
Requires person to meet the environment demands of needs, and safety of group members	Group promotes independence and capacity for self-direction through the support tasks and goals.
	Group promotes action flow and experience.
	Group contains occupational component as well as social component.
Permits subcortical centers to integrate and organize a response	Group focuses on the here-and-now group task, thus learning organization of input and output to sub-cortical centers of individuals.
	Group spontaneously involves members in the action.
Leads to self-reinforcement	Group members' support and feedback provides con-sensual validation for learning.
	Group builds on strengths.

*From 1978 Eleanor Clarke Slagle Lecture: Toward a science of adaptive responses. American Journal of Occu-pational Therapy 32(7): 429–437, by King, L. J. Copyright 1978 by the American Occupational Therapy Associa-tion, Inc. Reprinted with permission.

Adaptation is brought about through occupation or action. Thus, the func-tional group model is action-oriented: Members of the group are either directly involved in action or engaged in discussion about action. This orientation stems from the belief that behavior is a manifestation of the person as a whole, and in health, congruence between emotion and action is sought. This belief is based on the view that human beings are action-oriented and that "doing" is basic to their nature.

There are four types of action in the functional group model. First, action must be purposeful. The individuals and the group must recognize the activity be as congruent with their needs and goals (Box 4-10). Fidler and Fidler (1983) explain that "mastery and competence are verified and become obvious in the

---

Box 4-10
Purposeful Action in the Group

Mrs. Keil, recovering from a head injury, was ready to return to her family. However, in the cooking group, she could not find the utensils stored in the kitchen cabinets. Members suggested memory aids they have found useful. (Also see Tables 7-1, 8-1, 9-1.)

Box 4-11
Self-Initiated Action

On her next home visit, Mrs. Keil asked her husband to help her with reorganizing her kitchen.

reality of an end product. When the product resulting from an activity has social and cultural relevance to the individual and to his or her social groups, meaning is enhanced and social efficacy is affirmed" (p. 277). In addition, the activity must be suitable to the group members and their available skills. Finally, the human and nonhuman objects and environment related to the activity must be considered. Certain environments and objects may represent attitudes or feelings about one's degree of control, compliance, inclusion, or desirability. People grow from the natural, adaptive response to a proper fit between an individual and a group task. Fidler and Fidler (1983) explain, "When there is congruency between individual characteristics and the real and symbolic characteristics of an activity, there is greater likelihood that the doing experience will result in a feeling of pleasure and personal satisfaction, and that the essential learning will be integrated as an adaptive response" (p. 277).

Second, action in the functional group model must be self-initiated; that is, individuals must seek to improve their skills or understanding and seek a group on their own volition. If individuals do not personally choose to join or participate in the group, they will not achieve the goals they seek (Box 4-11).

Third, spontaneous, or here-and-now, action is essential; functional groups are based on experience, on experiential learning in the present. Through spontaneous actions, members can discover areas of behavior that interfere with adaptation. These groups provide a supportive environment, a place in which to practice living skills (Box 4-12). Rather than focusing on the past, the group provides a place for members to function in the present and practice skills in decision making, judgment, and perception, as well as in areas of special deficits. Through spontaneous action, learning in the present is emphasized. Fourth, action must be group-centered, a major distinguishing feature of the functional group. The

Box 4-12
Here-and-Now Action

Kristy expressed her frustration over the past week in her caregiver support group. Once again, she felt manipulated by her client. Through a role-playing situation, she explored various alternative ways of responding to prevent an angry outburst. (Also see Tables 7-1, 8-1, 9-1.)

group structure and goals always take into consideration the emotional and social needs of all members. The group leader aims to create an environment that
encourages interdependent action through consensus. Group-centered action allows maximal involvement through the interaction of all members—including
leaders—working toward a common goal and task. Through group-centered action, powerful forces that have important effects on members' sense of individual and group identity are mobilized (Box 4-13). These forces permit, enable, or
enhance self-initiated, purposeful, and spontaneous action.

A summary of the implications of the concepts forming the core of the functional group model follows. See Table 4-1 for the characteristics of adaptation
of the model, and see Boxes 4-14 to 4-17 for further assumptions concerning
functional groups.

Expected Results of Intervention

The goal of the functional group is to promote health or adaptation through purposeful, self-initiated, spontaneous, group-centered action. A group can have
multiple goals, thus incorporating the specific needs and goals of individual
members, as well as those more general goals and needs shared by all members.

The population served by the functional group is comprised of persons
with physical illness or injury, emotional disorders, congenital or developmental disabilities, or problems precipitated by the aging process, as well as individuals wishing to increase or maintain their level of adaptation and wellness.
The group can achieve specific goals in two categories: evaluation and the treatment process. First, the functional group provides an opportunity for observation and evaluation of behavior and interaction with the human and nonhuman environment for purposes of diagnosing performance problems. Second,
the functional group is structured to motivate members to act to achieve optimal function and adaptation, prevent occupational deficits, and maintain and
promote health and well-being.

Box 4-13
Group-Centered Action

In an after-school program for 7-year-olds, Joe was disruptive for the past few
weeks. He sought the attention of the leader, who was also Asian-American,
unlike the other group members. The leader decided to invite the group to talk
about this problem, acknowledging that everyone needs attention. She
suggested a sharing time at the end of the group, when everyone took a turn
sharing with the group. This, however, resulted in bedlam. After a brief talk
with members, sharing time was restructured to a game format, in which each
person was required to take a turn. (Also see Tables 7-1, 8-1, 9-1.)

Box 4-14
Social Systems Assumptions

We may make six statements about functional groups as social systems. That:

- Functional groups are not limited to therapy groups. As social systems they apply to naturally occurring groups in the community such as families or work groups.
- Functional groups provide a structure to guide the individual's participation. The structure and goals always address the social and emotional needs of the individual and are therefore said to be ego oriented.
- Groups intrinsically provide special therapeutic benefit, because occupational behavior is learned and shaped through a process of socialization.
- Functional group activities build on strengths of the individual in the group; therefore, there is interest in the strengths and weaknesses of each member.
- Functional groups can parallel and reflect the needs of the individual and the demands of society.
- Functional groups are assumed to provide benefits to members through mutual help. Groups are therefore structured so that members have the opportunity to help each other, thus enhancing members' perceptions and feelings of self-worth.

Box 4-15
Change Assumptions

We may make three statements about functional groups as agents of change. That:

- Groups can motivate people to action; functional groups are structured to motivate members to purposeful and meaningful action.
- Functional groups are experience-based groups, in which experiential learning occurs in the here and now. These groups provide a supportive environment, a place in which to practice living skills.
- Functional groups attempt to move members from dependence to independence or function and from maladaptation to adaptation.

> **Box 4-16**
> **Functional Orientation Assumptions**
>
> We may make three statements about the functional orientation of the functional group. That:
>
> - Functional groups provide a place for members to function in the reality of the present and practice skills in decision making, judgment, and perception, as well as in areas of special deficits.
> - Functional groups are concerned with elements of performance, as well as with types of performance, such as work, play, and self-maintenance.
> - Functional groups seek to build group cohesiveness; a certain degree of cohesiveness is necessary to achieve functional goals.

The functional group can be described as providing group experience in which:

- objects lead action
- action is used to enhance individual member's well-being and sense of internal control
- talking is used to clarify doing
- the therapist is teaching members to lead

The functional group may also be characterized by what it is not. First, it is not a leaderless group. The group leader plays an important role in facilitating the group process and planning for the group sessions. Second, it is not group psychotherapy. Although the functional group model is designed to provide therapy for patients with psychosocial problems, it does not focus on, nor is it primarily concerned with, developing insight through surfacing repressed or unconscious material. Third, it is not an activity therapy group. According to Slavson (1950), the founder of activity therapy, the goal of the activity therapy group is to bring about relief of "characterological" pathology (p. 2). The functional group seeks to enhance occupational behavior and thus adaptation. Fourth, the functional group is not focused on etiology. Thus, it does not seek to alter the etiology of a condition but rather facilitates change in the symptoms of a given condition as they interfere with occupation and adaptation. The emphasis is not on the diagnostic categories and symptoms: Because they are manifested in different ways in different individuals, the expectation of a particular set of symptoms may well impede the therapeutic progress for the group and the individual members.

Assessment Instruments

Methods of assessment are developed to collect data and information for determining whether certain problems exist and what intervention strategy to use

> ### Box 4-17
> ### Action Assumptions
>
> We may make four statements about the action component of the functional group. That:
>
> - The goal of the functional group is not the product of the group, even though the group may have a meaningful product, but rather that learning process that occurs through active participation.
> - Functional groups nurture interpersonal and intrapersonal development through activity choice, climate, and goals.
> - Functional groups make use of both the human and nonhuman environment and object relations. Attention is directed to attachments to people and objects, as well as to separations from people and objects.
> - Functional group leaders are cognizant of the individual's need for self-motivation and desire for mastery. They guide the activity of the group accordingly.

(Reed, 1984). The assessment instruments used in the functional group are discussed in Chapters 5 through 9. They include observation (verbal and nonverbal), content and process analysis, needs assessment, group protocol, observation guides for initial evaluation, and observation guides for assessing ongoing group function and structure (e.g., sociogram, member behavior rating forms, and group evaluation forms). In addition, group members are encouraged to be observers and evaluators in order to determine the validity of leader assessments.

Intervention Strategies

Intervention strategies are the media, modalities, methods, techniques, and equipment used to bring about change in the patient and achieve specific goals or objectives (Reed, 1984). Again, these strategies are detailed in Chapters 5 through 9 and include defining issues and expectations during the course of the group and using purposeful, self-initiated, spontaneous, group-centered action.

Logical Deductions

If the model is effective in bringing about change and achieving the stated goals, we can deduce certain results. The logical deductions are stated as hypotheses in question-or-answer form (Reed, 1984). If one implements the functional group model, we can expect the following results:

- group members' health needs will be met
- group members will learn the skills and occupational behaviors necessary for adaptation

Intervention Principles

According to Reed (1984), generalizations concerning the accuracy of a model must be derived from the results of tests of the hypotheses. These generalizations are the intervention principles. The functional group model is based primarily on empirical evidence, and this stage is not yet complete. As with all models, as information becomes available, and the context of practice changes, new questions should be raised. At present, we can say that there is continually strong growing evidence in the occupational therapy and related literature to support our hypotheses that go beyond the four studies originally cited (Henry, Nelson, and Duncombe, 1984; Mumford, 1974; Odhner, 1970; Schwartzberg, Howe, and McDermott, 1982). Furthermore, the functional group has been recognized as a model applied to practice and theoretical discussions (Barnes and Schwartzberg, in press; Barnes and Schwartzberg, 1999; Borg and Bruce, 1991; Bruce, 1988; Cole, 1993; Kaplan, 1988; Kielhofner, 1992; Posthuma, 1989; Schwartzberg, 1993, 1998, 1999; Schwartzberg and Abeles, 1991; Steffan, 1990), as well as a model used as a basis for research (Clark et al., 1997; Jackson et al., 1998; Mandel et al., 1999). The relevant research and applications, as well as pertinent analyses of the model (Kielhofner, 1992), will be discussed in Chapter 10.

Conclusion

The functional group model is an occupational therapy approach to group work and the first comprehensive model of the profession's group practice. It is based in part on the work of practitioners and researchers in the decades preceding the book's original 1986 publication of the model and in part on the recognition of recent needs in the field of occupational therapy. The framework presented serves as a guide; answers posed to new or difficult questions can be measured against the statements in the relevant categories. It is expected that verification of the model will continue in the future.

Review Questions

1. Why is the early literature on group dynamics important to the understanding of the functional group model? What are some of the principles of group dynamics?
2. What is meant by adaptation and how does the functional group model propose to effect adaptation?
3. What are four types of action basic to the functional group model?
4. If a functional group meets the needs and goals of the group can it also meet the needs of the individual group members?

References

Bales, R. F. (1950). Interaction Process Analysis: A Method for the Study of Small Groups. Cambridge, MA: Addison-Wesley.

Barnes, M. A., and Schwartzberg, S. L. (in press). Activity analysis of group process. Journal of Psychotherapy in Independent Practice.

Barnes, M. A., and Schwartzberg, S. L. (1999). A case in study: An occupational therapy approach. In S. Simon Fehr (ed.), Introduction to Group Therapy: A Practical Guide for the Future Group Leader. Binghamton, NY: The Haworth Press.

Barris, R., Kielhofner, G., and Hawkins, J. H. (1983). Psychosocial Occupational Therapy: Practice in a Pluralistic Arena. Laurel, MD: Ramsco.

Benne, K. D., and Sheats, P. (1978). Functional roles of group members. In L. P. Bradford (ed.), Group Development (2nd ed.), pp. 52–61. La Jolla, CA: University Associates.

Bennis, W. B., and Shepard, H. A. (1956). A theory of group development. Human Relations 9(4): 415–457.

Borg, B., and Bruce, M. A. (1991). The Group System: The Therapeutic Activity Group in Occupational Therapy. Thorofare, NJ: Slack.

Bruce, M. A. (1988). Occupational therapy in group treatment. In D. W. Scott and N. Katz (eds.), Occupational Therapy in Mental Health: Principles in Practice, pp. 116–132. Philadelphia: Taylor & Francis.

Burke, J. P. (1983). Defining occupation: Importing and organizing interdisciplinary knowledge. In G. Kielhofner (ed.), Health Through Occupation: Theory and Practice in Occupational Therapy, pp. 125–138. Philadelphia: F. A. Davis.

Cartwright, D., and Zander, A. (eds.) (1968). Group Dynamics Research and Theory (3rd ed.). New York: Harper & Row.

Clark, F., Azen, S. P., Zemke, R., Jackson, J., Carlson, M., Mandel, D., Hay, J., Josephson, K., Cherry, B., Hessel, C., Palmer, J., and Lipson, L. (1997). Occupational therapy for independent-living older adults: A randomized controlled trial. Journal of the American Medical Association 278: 1321–1326.

Cole, M. B. (1993). Group Dynamics. In Occupational Therapy: The Theoretical Basis and Practice Application of Group Treatment. Thorofare, NJ: Slack.

Csikszentmihalyi, M. (1975). Beyond Boredom and Anxiety: The Experience of Play in Work and Games. San Francisco: Jossey-Bass.

Csikszentmihalyi, M. (1990). Flow: The Psychology of Optimal Experience. New York: Harper Collins Publishers.

Fidler, G. S., and Fidler, J. W. (1978). Doing and becoming: Purposeful action and self-actualization. American Journal of Occupational Therapy 32(5): 305–310.

Fidler, G. S., and Fidler, J. W. (1983). Doing and becoming: The occupational therapy experience. In G. Kielhofner (ed.), Health Through Occupation: Theory and Practice in Occupational Therapy, pp. 267–280. Philadelphia: F. A. Davis.

Garland, J. A., Jones, H. E., and Kolodny, R. (1965). A Model for Stages of Development in Social Work. Boston: Boston University School of Social Work.

Henry, A. D., Nelson, D. L., and Duncombe, L. W. (1984). Choice making in group and individual activity. American Journal of Occupational Therapy 38(4): 245–251.

Jackson, J., Carlson, M., Mandel, D., Zemke, R., and Clark, F. (1998). Occupation in lifestyle redesign: The well elderly study occupational therapy program. American Journal of Occupational Therapy 52(5): 326–336.

Kaplan, K. L. (1988). Directive Group Therapy: Innovative Mental Health Treatment. Thorofare, NJ: Slack.

Kielhofner, G. (1992). Conceptual Foundations of Occupational Therapy. Philadelphia: F. A. Davis.

King, L. J. (1978). 1978 Eleanor Clarke Slagle Lecture: Toward a science of adaptive responses. American Journal of Occupational Therapy 32(7): 429–437.

Knowles, M., and Knowles, H. (1972). Introduction to Group Dynamics (rev. ed.). New York: Association Press.

Lifton, W. M. (1961). Working with Groups: Group Process and Individual Growth. New York: John Wiley & Sons.

Mandel, D. R., Jackson, J. M., Zemke, R., Nelson, L., & Clark, F. A. (1999). Lifestyle Redesign Implementing the Well Elderly Program. Bethesda, MD: American Occupational Therapy Association.

Maslow, A. H. (1970). Motivation and Personality (2nd ed.). New York: Harper & Row.

Mosey, A. C. (1973). Meeting health needs. American Journal of Occupational Therapy 27(1): 14–17.

Mumford, M. S. (1974). A comparison of interpersonal skills in verbal and activity groups. American Journal of Occupational Therapy 28(5): 281–283.

Odhner, F. (1970). A study of group tasks as facilitators of verbalization among hospitalized schizophrenic patients. American Journal of Occupational Therapy 24(1): 7–12.

Posthuma, B. W. (1989). Small Groups in Therapy Settings: Process and Leadership. Boston: Little, Brown & Company.

Reed, K. L. (1984). Models of Practice in Occupational Therapy. Baltimore: Williams & Wilkins.

Reed, K. L., and Sanderson, S. (1983). Concepts of Occupational Therapy (2nd ed.). Baltimore: Williams & Wilkins.

Schwartzberg, S. L. (1999). The use of groups in the rehabilitation of persons with head injury and the reasoning skills employed by the group facilitator. In C. A. Unsworth (ed.), Cognitive and Perceptual Disorders A Clinical Reasoning Approach to Evaluation and Intervention. Philadelphia: F. A. Davis.

Schwartzberg, S. L. (1998). Group Process. In M. E. Neistadt and E. B. Crepeau (eds.), Willard and Spackman's Occupational Therapy (9th ed.), pp. 120-131. Philadelphia: J. B. Lippincott.

Schwartzberg, S. L. (1993). Tools of practice, section 2: Group process. In H. L. Hopkins and H. D. Smith (eds.), Willard and Spackman's Occupational Therapy (8th ed.), pp. 275–280. Philadelphia: J. B. Lippincott.

Schwartzberg, S. L., and Abeles, J. (1991). Occupational therapy. In L. I. Sederer (ed.), Inpatient Psychiatry: Diagnosis and Treatment (3rd ed.), pp. 298–319. Baltimore: Williams & Wilkins.

Schwartzberg, S. L., Howe, M. C., and McDermott, A. (1982). A comparison of three treatment group formats for facilitating social interaction. Occupational Therapy in Mental Health 2(4): 1–16.

Slavson, S. R. (1950). Analytic Group Psychotherapy With Children, Adolescents and Adults. New York: Columbia University Press.

Steffan, J. A. (1990). Productive occupation in small task groups of adults: Synthesis and annotations of the social psychology literature. In A. C. Bundy, N. D. Prendergast, J. A. Steffan, and D. Thorn (eds.), Review of Selected Literature on Occupation and Health, pp. 175–281. Rockville, MD: American Occupational Therapy Association.

Tuckman, B. W. (1965). Developmental sequence in small groups. Psychological Bulletin 63: 384–399.

White, R. W. (1959). Motivation reconsidered: The concept of competence. The Psychological Review 66: 297–333.

White, R. W. (1971). The urge towards competence. American Journal of Occupational Therapy 25(6): 271–274.

Yalom, I. D. (1970). The Theory and Practice of Group Psychotherapy. New York: Basic Books.

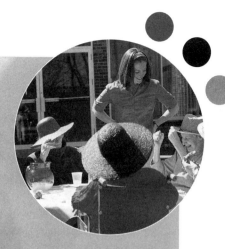

Part II
Leadership and Four Stages of the Functional Group

Part I dealt primarily with definitions of groups and descriptions of how they function. We examined occupational therapy group work from the perspective of history and of current practice. Finally, a functional model for group work was presented.

In Part II, we consider the application of the functional group model to clinical practice. Chapter 5 is an overview of the issues and expectations concerning group leadership, followed by an exploration of the skills required for effective group leadership and a discussion of intervention strategies intended to assist group leaders.

The leader can better assist the group to achieve its goals if the leader is aware of the stages of a group's development, the inevitable critical events, and the problems usually raised and solved. The developmental stages through which a group must travel do not always proceed in a predictable manner. The course is often marked with fluctuations. Stages may overlap, or the group may temporarily regress to earlier stages. A group may also stay on a plateau for numerous sessions before moving to a different level of function. Understanding patterns of change enables the leader to guide the group and assist the members to mobilize their resources toward achieving both individual and group goals.

Although patterns in the development of a group may often continue over a number of sessions, each group meeting will also display developmental characteristics. Each group meeting can be seen as a microcosm of a sequence of meetings. An individual group session will begin with a formation period, when members greet each other, establish the climate, and review or establish the goals and norms of the group. The session then proceeds to the working stage and eventually enters the termination period. Short-term and open groups go through a developmental pattern in individual sessions, even though these developmental periods may be abbreviated and more superficial than in the long-term groups.

Chapters 6 through 9 follow the developmental sequence of groups from beginning to end. Chapter 6 introduces the first phase of the functional group, the design stage. The issues and expectations typically found in the second, or formation, stage are discussed in Chapter 7. Chapter 8 presents the important issues and expectations of the third phase, the development stage. Chapter 9 covers the fourth phase, the termination stage. At each point, leader functions and intervention strategies are discussed. In addition, we introduce in Chapter 6 detailed case studies of two sample groups. We will follow these groups through each of the four stages to enable the reader to view the results of applying the functional group model.

Chapter 5
Role of the Leader in the Functional Group

Sometimes it is merely the offering of help which is therapeutic.
(ROGERS, 1967, P. 270)

Definitions of Leadership

Social scientists have long been interested in the subject of group leadership, and much research has been done on the topic. Researchers have been concerned with identifying characteristics that make individuals effective group leaders. In approaching this issue, social scientists accepted a number of diverse assumptions about leadership; consequently, their studies led them in different directions. In the following pages, we will discuss four attempts to define leadership.

Personality Traits

For many years, researchers viewed leadership as the combination of personality traits in a particular person. They studied particularly the traits that they believed a good leader should possess: intelligence, warmth, decisiveness, and assertiveness.

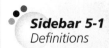

Sidebar 5-1
Definitions

Leadership: *The ability to promote those behaviors that lead to the satisfaction of group needs*

Traits of a good leader: *Features such as intelligence, warmth, decisiveness, and assertiveness*

Situations: *A particular set of group circumstances that determines how a leader will behave*

Behaviors: *The ways in which group members react to a particular pattern or style of leadership*

Functions: *The ways in which the leader helps the group achieve its goals and strengthen itself*

This approach yielded little conclusive evidence. There were inevitably good leaders who were not decisive, warm, or assertive although these traits were found to be common among people who were judged to be effective leaders. This direction of inquiry also proved futile in identifying prospective leaders. Nevertheless, the research results did suggest, according to Stogdill (1948), "that leadership is a relation that exists between persons in a social situation, and that persons who are leaders in one situation may not necessarily be leaders in other situations" (p. 65).

Situations

When research into personality traits failed to provide conclusive data, social scientists turned to studying the circumstances in which leadership was present. They asked, do leaders emerge from a particular set of group circumstances? The hypothesis was that a leader's behavior in one setting may differ from that of a second leader in a different setting. In addition, social scientists postulated that the behavior of a leader might differ from one group situation to another. Homans (1950) pursued this course of inquiry by studying groups on a naval vessel during wartime. He found that leaders among these individuals changed according to the demands of the situation at hand. When there was little work to be done on board ship and groups faced inactivity and boredom, individuals who could be entertaining became popular and won recognition. When the ship came to port, those who had knowledge about the port, had been there before, or had contacts on land immediately became the leaders of the group. This study seems to emphasize that groups select leaders according to how well an individual's skill or knowledge meets the needs of the situation (Box 5-1).

Behaviors

A different approach to the study of leadership was conceived by Lewin, Lippitt, and White (1939), who examined the effects that different leadership behaviors have on groups of 10-year-old boys in a summer day camp. The ex-

> **Box 5-1**
> **Born Leaders?**
>
> Similar to the earlier emphasis on personality traits, the situation and timing imply that leadership is more a matter of chance than a skill that can be learned and developed.

periment studied three different leadership styles: autocratic, democratic, and laissez-faire. Group leaders were trained to assume these different leadership styles. In the autocratic group, the decision-making power was under the control of the designated leader. In the democratic group, the decision-making power was in the control of the group, but under the guidance of the leader; in the laissez-faire group, the decision-making power was left entirely to the individuals in the group.

The autocratic leader dictated rules to be followed and did not discuss problems with the children. He did not participate in the group except when giving instructions and demonstrating how the instructions should be followed. Under democratic leadership, all policies were open for discussion and decision by the group. The leader helped the group to build a decision-making process of its own. The leader acted as a resource person for the group. The laissez-faire leader presented the group members with the supplies that they needed for their work and gave them information when asked. Otherwise, this leader took no part in the group. Lewin reached five conclusions after evaluating these three groups:

1. The democratic leadership style resulted in a more satisfying, efficient leadership than did the laissez-faire.
2. Autocratic leadership resulted in a slightly higher group productivity than did the other two leadership styles but showed a significantly poorer quality of work than did the group with democratic leadership.
3. The autocratic leadership style created hostility and aggression in the group members.
4. There was greater dependency and less individuality in the autocratically led group than in the democratic group.
5. A greater degree of group cohesiveness, a sense of comradeship, and a high morale were seen more in the democratic group than in either of the other two groups.

These studies were published by Lewin, Lippitt, and White (1939) and have now become classic (Box 5-2).

Functions

According to another group of researchers, leadership functions are directly related to group functions (Box 5-3). There are two categories of leadership function. The first relates to the achievement of the group goals or tasks and is called

> ### Box 5-2
> ### Influential Patterns
>
> The results of research by Lewin, Lippitt, and White show clearly that different patterns of leadership result in different kinds of behavior among members of a group. They identified three distinct types of leadership styles:
>
> - Democratic
> - Laissez-faire
> - Autocratic

the task function. The second relates to helping the group build and maintain a process that enables the group to strengthen itself. This is called the maintenance function. In successful groups, both task and maintenance functions are part of the ongoing life of the group. Group behavior may address both of these functions simultaneously, but frequently one function is served at the expense of the other. For example, a group may be so intent on reaching the task goal that it does not strengthen its decision-making process and depends on one individual (perhaps the leader) to make all decisions. In this case, the group is putting its efforts into task functions while neglecting its maintenance functions. The relative importance of group building (maintenance) and goal achievement (task) for any group may change dramatically from the early meetings to the later stages of development.

In most group situations, one person is designated the leader (Box 5-4).

Lippitt developed a list of ways in which the group leader can increase the effectiveness of the group (1961, p. 35):

- At the beginning of any group's life, help the group come to a clear understanding of the goals that it wants to reach.
- Help the group become aware of its own procedures.
- Help the group understand the skills, talents, and resources within its own membership.
- Help the group develop group methods of evaluation so that both leader and members can find ways of improving their procedures.

> ### Box 5-3
> ### Relationship to Group
>
> Leadership is viewed as the ability to promote those behaviors that lead to the satisfaction of group needs.

> **Box 5-4**
> **Responsibility Is Shared**
>
> The leader needs to share leadership responsibility with the members so that they can learn both maintenance and task functions.

- Help the group learn to accept new ideas and members without conflict.
- Assist the group in creating new tasks and terminating outdated ones.

Many of the suggestions presented by Lippitt (1961) strongly resemble the conduct found in the democratic leadership style (Box 5-5).

Our understanding of the group leader's role has changed over time and will continue to change as research and practical experiences modify our views of leadership. As leaders of functional groups, we understand the leader to be in a dynamic relationship with the members. This calls on the clinical reasoning skills and related actions of the leader. In this context, the emphasis is on what actions are required by the group members, under various conditions, if they are to achieve their goals, and on how group members can best take part in these actions. When leadership is defined in terms of behaviors that further the goals of the group, it becomes difficult to separate leadership roles from membership roles. Groups with a highly structured, leader-centered process will have low membership involvement. Groups with an emphasis on membership involvement will have less leadership involvement. Tannenbaum and Schmidt (1958) identified the range of possible leader and member involvement on a continuum ranging from leader-centered leadership to group-centered leadership (Fig. 5-1).

Working with informal groups in the community such as family or peer groups may require a different leadership from that in a more structured group. The leadership role may be closer to the role of a consultant, an educator, or a resource person. In such cases, leader interaction with group members may be limited and defined by the situation.

The theory that leadership varies according to the leader's interaction with the group is congruent with the model for the functional group in occupational therapy. This concept of leadership encourages the would-be leader to develop the

> **Box 5-5**
> **Synergistic Process**
>
> The role of the leader is to develop and support the processes within the group that enable members to grow and take on greater responsibility for making decisions and for reaching group goals.

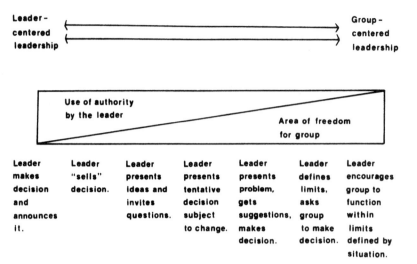

Figure 5-1. Leader–member continuum. (Modified from Tannenbaum, R., and Schmidt, W. H. [1958]. How to choose a leadership pattern. Harvard Business Review 36 [March–April]:96.)

skills necessary for active participation in group functions and the ability to assume a variety of leadership roles. Interpersonal effectiveness is a measure of the degree to which one's leadership behavior matches one's intended role as group leader.

Leadership Skills

Planning the Group Activity

The group leader is responsible for planning the activity of the functional group. In the early sessions of a closed or ongoing group, the leader must select the group task and decide the length, number, and types of tasks in each meeting. As soon as possible, the leader must begin involving members in selecting tasks and teaching members to assist in formulating and adapting the goals of the group's activity.

In the process of choosing an activity, the leader relies on his or her professional knowledge of activities. Hopkins, Smith, and Tiffany (1983) published guidelines on selecting occupational therapy activities for individual patients, and these guidelines can be applied to functional groups. In selecting a group activity, the leader must bear in mind the following main points:

- The goals of the activity should have meaning for the group members. The meaning of any activity will vary, depending on the stages of development of the group. The activity should be useful to individual members and related to their interests and roles.
- The group members should be able to participate in choosing or adapting the given activity, thus assuring a minimum level of self-initiated mental or physical participation in the process.
- The task should enable members to take an active role in the group. They

should be interested in the task; the demands of the task should elicit an adaptive response, and the members' response should be supported by its organization at the subcortical level.

- The activity should be adaptable and assessable according to member skills, ages, or performance levels. This includes an awareness of the individual's relationship to and role in the group.

The task may be recreational, physical, academic, or vocational (Fig. 5-2), but regardless of its nature, the task must facilitate the attainment of group goals, as well as individual treatment goals (Box 5-6). Group discussion is an activity common to practically all group meetings, but the leader, in consultation with the group, must decide how much time is to be spent in discussion and how much is to be spent on the task itself.

Members of therapy groups often have a limited repertoire of social skills and interests. In the past, they may have often met with failure when attempting new tasks, and this failure discouraged their involvement in new experiences. Because of this tendency, the group leader must not only plan the activity but also stimulate member interest in the task.

Genuineness and Empathy

A genuine person is one who can be himself or herself while interacting with other people and maintain an openness to the feelings and attitudes that are experienced. This general principle applies to a group leader. The term genuineness implies an ability to share intimate feelings when appropriate. The leader is conscious of the feelings he or she is experiencing and is able to communi-

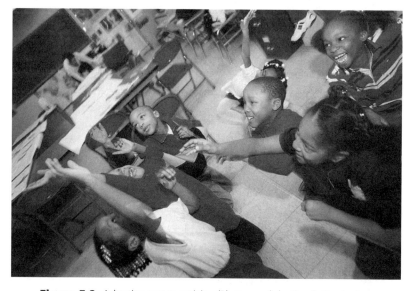

Figure 5-2. Adaptive group activity. (Photograph by Sarah Brezinsky.)

Box 5-6
Careful Selection

The task is a crucial factor in the treatment of individuals in a functional group. The leader considers the following attributes in selecting a group task:

- Activity goals must be meaningful to group members
- Group members should participate in task selection
- The task should encourage members to be active
- The task should be able to be graded and adaptable

cate them to the group members, if desired. In studying therapy groups, Galigor (1977) found that group members who view their leader as "open, accepting, responsive, and confident" did not drop out of the groups as readily as did those members who saw their leader as "distant, neutral or professional."

Egan (1975) identifies two characteristics of the genuine person. The first is spontaneity; the genuine person is able to communicate easily about immediate events without being impulsive. When the leader reflects on what has been said in the group, he or she is motivated by a concern for the group members, not by self-protection. The second characteristic of the genuine person is non-defensiveness. "The genuine person is non-defensive. He has a feeling for his areas of strength and his areas of deficit in living and presumably is trying to live more effectively all the time. When a client expresses negative attitudes toward him, he tries to understand what the client is thinking and feeling, and he continues to work with him" (p. 92).

Empathy, often explained as caring for and understanding another individual, is another skill of the effective group leader (Box 5-7). In a factor analysis of the attributes of good leaders, Lieberman, Yalom, and Miles (1973) found that the most effective leaders were rated high in caring. They defined caring as a leadership style that offered members protection, friendship, and affection. Caring leaders provided frequent opportunities for members to receive feedback, as well as praise and encouragement for their behavior. Another quality

Box 5-7
Honed Skills

The effective group leader has honed several skills, among them:

- Genuineness, which includes spontaneity and nondefensiveness, and
- Empathy, a strong sense of caring that includes feedback and communication.

of caring was careful listening and attending to what was being expressed in the group. Members are reassured when the speaker identifies himself or herself with the listener's problems and accepts the other person's emotional reactions at face value. Communication that conveys respect for the listener is supportive and reduces the defensiveness of the listener. Gestures and other behavioral signs are also important in communicating empathy and caring.

Modeling Behavior

In Chapter 1, we discussed how the structure of the group helps to establish the legitimate group norms, values, and limits of behavior. The group leader has a role in this process, particularly in the early stages of the group (Box 5-8). The functional group leader helps members learn new behaviors that will increase their ability to meet group needs and personal goals. This learning process can occur in a number of different ways, through direct instruction, through group experiences, or through a combination of both.

The studies of Lieberman, Yalom, and Miles (1973) found that effective group leaders were characterized by the term "meaning attribution." The term refers to the tendency of the group leader to clarify, explain, understand, and interpret what is happening in the group. These points in a discussion give members a framework for change. The authors found that effective leaders spent time in their groups explaining to the members why they did what they did and why they structured the group in a particular way. They also shared with the group their perceptions of how members interacted with each other at specific moments during the group session. Napier and Gershenfeld (1973) also support the importance of meaning attribution to group learning. They comment, "Learning is more likely to be retained and internalized in an atmosphere in which leaders (or other members) clarify what they or others are doing" (p. 34).

A second approach to teaching new skills is through the modeling of the desired behaviors (Box 5-9). According to the social learning theory of Bandura (1969), this is a valuable method for learning and teaching new skills. To teach group members through modeling, leaders must first learn the behavior that they hope members will learn as part of their group experience. Johnson (1972) writes, "The word modeling refers to the process by which one person engages in ideal behavior to serve as an example to be imitated by other persons. If you, for example, engage in self-disclosure and the other person imitates you by also engaging in self-disclosure, a modeling process has taken place" (p. 189).

Box 5-8
Position of Strength

The leader is viewed as the central person or spokesperson of the group, and his or her overt behavior strengthens the norms and values of the group.

> **Box 5-9**
> **Model Behavior**
>
> The imitation of leader behavior is followed by a positive reinforcement of group members through recognition and approval.

A group member who is relatively unskilled in interpersonal relations may learn interpersonal skills by observing the leader-model. If a group member is brought to note the consequences of any particular behavior, the member will see that positive results can be achieved by adapting his or her particular mode of conduct. In another instance, a member may know a certain mode of behavior but not know when to apply it; the leader can guide the member in discovering the correct circumstances for certain modes of behavior. In perhaps the most common scenario, a group member simply watches and copies the leader's behavior. For this reason, leaders must carefully consider the modes of conduct and the responses they will elicit from the group.

According to Johnson (1972), a leader must understand the following aspects of the modeling process to teach a certain mode of behavior effectively:

- You must have the attention of the other person. If the other person is not aware of your behavior, he or she cannot imitate it.
- If others think that imitating your behavior will help them to accomplish their own goals, they will be apt to imitate your behavior.
- If imitating leader behavior brought success in the past, there is a stronger possibility that leader behavior will be imitated in the present.
- If other people value your friendship, like you, or seek your approval, they are more likely to imitate your behavior.
- People are more likely to imitate your behavior when they are emotionally aroused.
- If another person is unsure about what behavior is appropriate in a given situation and you are not unsure, that person will tend to imitate you.

Leaders who wish to help a member develop interpersonal skills must demonstrate those skills in the group. Further, they must develop a group climate that is supportive and accepting so that members will dare to try new behaviors in the group. Group members make the most progress in a group in which they feel comfortable and are encouraged to explore new possibilities.

Reality Testing

The effective leader also assists the group to achieve its goals through reality testing. The shared reality that is part of each functional group meeting creates opportunities for testing reality (Box 5-10). Further, because of its norms and its support for honest expression, the group offers ample opportunities for con-

---

Box 5-10
Therapeutic Milieu

Because of its focus on a task and on the relationship between thinking and feeling, the functional group provides an excellent milieu for learning new behaviors.

---

sensual validation. Consensual validation is achieved through a comparison of one's own interpersonal evaluations with those of others in the group. Here, perceptions can be tested and discussed. Here, behavior can be altered or reinforced according to its relation to reality. Recording the group session on audiotape or videotape and replaying the tapes in the group can enhance reality testing.

In a list of curative factors present in therapy groups, Yalom (1970) places reality testing near the top of the list. Similarly, Carl Rogers (1959) includes reality testing among patient behaviors that reflect a good therapeutic relationship.

In addition to assisting members to test the reality of their behaviors, the leader should test the reality of his or her behavior within the group. Leaders often become the target of members' conflictual behaviors regarding persons in authority. This involves a phenomenon called transference. In transference, the member finds in the leader certain qualities associated with past figures of authority. Usually the leader does not actually possess these qualities. The effective leader can counter these inaccurate perceptions through reality testing and can do much to clarify a member's perception of the leader as an individual.

Communicating

The interpersonal effectiveness of the leader depends on his or her ability to communicate clearly, create the desired impression, and influence another person in a specific manner. Interpersonal effectiveness can be improved through several techniques, including self-disclosure, feedback on behavior, and adjustment of behavior until other individuals perceive it as it was intended. In this section we will discuss five of the most commonly used communication skills.

Listening and Responding

The way you listen and respond to another person is crucial for building a positive relationship. Through how you listen and respond, you can make the relationship either a distant one or a close, more personal one. In a close relationship, it is important to let the other person know that you have heard and understood what was said to you.

According to Johnson (1972), one of the major barriers to building close relationships is the tendency to judge, evaluate, approve, or disapprove of a statement that has been made to you. "This happens when the sender makes a statement and you respond internally or openly with, 'I think you're wrong,' 'I

don't like what you said,' 'I think your views are right,' or 'I agree entirely.' "
(p. 75). People tend to respond with evaluative statements when strong feelings
are involved. The stronger the feelings, the more likely that those involved will
evaluate the statements according to their own points of view.

Learning to be a good listener is an important skill for every group leader.
It takes considerable effort and practice to learn to listen accurately. Below are
four suggestions for improving listening skills.

- Make a firm commitment to listen.
- Get physically ready to listen and attend.
- Dismiss other concerns from your mind. Concentrate on the other person
  as a communicator.
- Give the person a full hearing, avoiding interruption unless absolutely nec-
  essary. Impatience can lead to false understanding.

Feedback

Stating your reaction to another person's behavior is called feedback. The purpose of this technique is to help other people become aware of how you perceive their behavior and how their behavior affects you (Box 5-11).

Feedback should be given in a manner that is not threatening to the other
person. The more defensive individuals are, the less likely they will correctly
hear and understand your remarks. People need both positive and negative
feedback. They need to know not only what is ineffective but also what is effective so that they can correct the one and continue the other. Feedback is most
successfully communicated when a relationship of trust and confidence has
been established in the group.

Timing is important in giving and receiving feedback. It is generally most
helpful if it is connected with a specific incident; that is, if it can be given in
terms of objective data that have just been observed in the group. This gives the
recipient of the feedback the opportunity to compare it with the reactions or
observations of the other members in the group. Sometimes, it is unwise to give
feedback right after the incident in question, particularly if strong feelings have
been aroused and people need time to calm down. Negative feedback is often
viewed as criticism, and people react to it by defending themselves through ra-
tionalization, denial, or suspicion of the motives of the person giving the feedback. Therefore, a leader or member should exercise discretion when giving
negative feedback.

Box 5-11
Reaching Goals

Feedback and timing enable people to improve performance in achieving their
desired goals.

Feedback can be given to a group, as well as to individuals. Like individuals, a group can benefit from receiving information about its performance. The group may need to know that the atmosphere is defensive, that members are having difficulty being heard, or that there is too much reliance on the leader. The general guidelines for individual feedback also apply to group feedback. The group may receive feedback from members acting as participant observers or leaders. Forms and questionnaires may be used to elicit feedback.

Concreteness

In some groups, vagueness and superficiality can become a serious problem, leading members to avoid talking about specific issues. The leader can help the group move toward its goals by using concrete language to communicate with the group. If leaders use concrete examples in their communications with the group members, the members, by imitation, will learn to focus on concrete behaviors in their explorations of their own behavior patterns. Learning to be concrete can be particularly helpful to members of functional groups in which avoidance and reality contact have been identified as problems for certain members.

Successful problem solving requires becoming progressively more concrete. When a group is involved in problem-solving tasks, a problem concretely stated can more easily be translated into achieved goals. If goals are stated in concrete terms, members can begin to define the means needed to reach those goals. Further, concrete goals can be broken down into smaller, more easily achieved subunits. Finally, concreteness can be effectively used to reduce ambiguity, and when ambiguity is lessened, the anxiety of group members is also lessened.

Confrontation

Johnson (1972) defines confrontation as "a deliberate attempt to help another person examine the consequences of some aspect of his behavior. It is an invitation to self-examination" (p. 160). He continues:

> "A confrontation originates from a desire on the part of the confronter to involve himself more deeply with the person he is confronting. Confrontation is a way of expressing concern for another person and a wish to increase the mutual involvement in the relationship. The first rule of confrontation is, "'Do not confront another person if you do not intend to increase your involvement with him.'" (p. 160)

The decision to confront another person is made on the basis of one's relationship with that person. The quality of the relationship is important; the stronger the relationship, the more powerful the confrontation will be. If that person's motivation to change is low or if his or her anxiety level is high, the confrontation will probably be seen not as an invitation for self-examination but as an attack. In this instance, a confrontation should not be initiated (Box 5-12).

In their study of therapy groups, Lieberman, Yalom, and Miles (1973) found four attributes of effective leaders; among these was moderation in the area of emotional stimulation. By emotional stimulation, these authors meant

> **Box 5-12**
> **Sensitivity Required**
>
> A leader must consider the ability of the person being confronted to act on the confrontation.

behaviors that strongly encourage revealing feelings. Self-disclosure and confrontation may encourage and sometimes coerce members to go beyond a level that they feel is comfortable for them. This may cause members to withdraw or even to leave the group. Under most circumstances, confrontation is best approached tentatively and with qualifications that enable the member to accept the message, add to it, or receive it without feeling accused by the leader. Confrontation is best done in a group that has achieved a high degree of trust and cohesiveness.

Self-Disclosure

Letting another person know what you think, feel, or want is called self-disclosure. The term refers to revealing feelings about a present situation and giving information about the past that is relevant to an understanding of how you experience the present. Leaders who practice self-disclosure are more easily seen by members as real people rather than as impersonal leaders (Box 5-13). The past history is helpful only if it clarifies why the leader is reacting in a particular way. Engaging in self-disclosure means taking a risk of being misunderstood or rejected; therefore, in responding to another person's self-disclosure, it is important to be accepting and supportive. Jourard (1964) has studied self-disclosure extensively. He reports that women seem to find self-disclosure easier than men and that some cultural groups are more prone to self-disclosure than others.

Leadership Strategies

The several leadership skills just described enable the leader of a group to guide members in their efforts to achieve specific goals. In addition to employing specific leadership skills, a leader may use strategies designed to gather information from an entire group (Box 5-14). Each strategy uses the same three-step

> **Box 5-13**
> **Judicious Disclosure**
>
> Members get to know and understand leaders not through past history but through knowing how they react in present situations.

> **Box 5-14**
> **Three-Step Strategy**
>
> A leader's information-gathering strategies include getting information from the group, reporting data to the members, and having them identify the problem and devise a solution.

process. First, the leader collects data about the group. Second, the leader reports the data to the group. Finally, the group defines the problem indicated by the data and designs a solution. Bradford, Stock, and Horwitz (1978) insist that both members and leaders—that is, the entire group—must collaborate in all parts of this process. In the functional group, the leader is responsible for teaching group members how to participate in procedures. As observers and resource persons, the leaders can offer specific concerns for discussion, gathered from observation, analysis, and experience.

A leader can also teach group members to assume some of the data-gathering functions. Leaders can use several techniques for gathering observations about a group's verbal and nonverbal behavior. A description of several of these follows, and they can be used in conjunction with the leadership skills already discussed.

Methods of Observation

Sociogram

A sociogram is an instrument that provides data on a communication pattern in the group. It charts specifically who talks to whom. By using this technique, the observer can follow the flow of the conversation and identify members who speak often, members who speak seldom, and members who receive comments or questions.

To use a sociogram, the leader draws a circle and marks the members of the group by name in their places in the circle (Fig. 5-3). The leader then draws a line for each statement or question, indicating the initiator and the recipient. A sociogram usually records the number of statements made during a 10-minute period. Some lines may extend only to the center of the circle; these represent statements that were made to the group as a whole and that were not directed toward a specific individual. The arrows at both ends of the line indicate that the recipient responded to the statement. In the sample in Figure 5-3, Bruce received more statements than anyone else; Mary spoke to two persons, but no one responded to her or addressed a statement to her. Although 15 statements were made during that 10-minute period, Jeff was not involved in any of these communications.

Sociograms are commonly used at intervals during the course of a group meeting (Box 5-15). Sociograms are also useful in identifying group members' communication patterns. For instance, a sociogram may reveal that some group

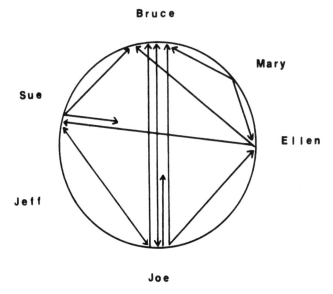

Bruce

Mary

Sue

Ellen

Jeff

Joe

Figure 5-3. Sociogram.

members talked only to the leader, perhaps indicating their dependence on the leader and their reluctance or inability to get involved with the other group members.

Interaction Process Analysis

Bales (1950) developed a method for analyzing verbal interactions made during a group meeting (Fig. 5-4). His system for observing and recording is based on his theory regarding the two main points of group process: task issues and maintenance issues. Bales sought to distinguish between communications that give information and those that seek information. He also differentiated between emotionally negative and positive expressions and between behavior and verbal content. This system of communication analysis can be added to the sociogram by marking the lines of the sociogram with letters keyed to Bales's categories, thereby recording both who talks to whom and the types of communications made.

Box 5-15
Gathering Data

Schwartzberg, Howe, and McDermott (1982) report doing a sociogram for 5 minutes at two different points in the group session, at 20 minutes and again at 40 minutes after the beginning of the group session, to gather research data on group communication.

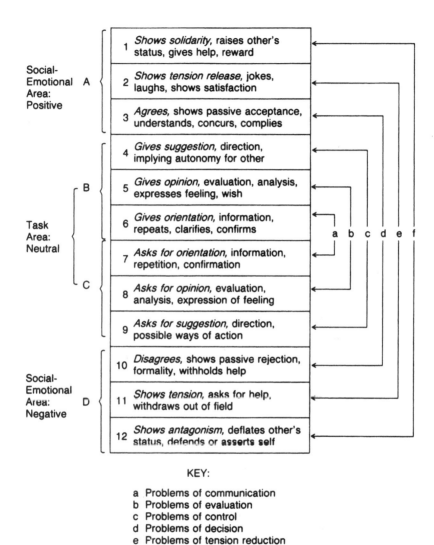

KEY:

a Problems of communication
b Problems of evaluation
c Problems of control
d Problems of decision
e Problems of tension reduction
f Problems of reintegration

A Positive reactions
B Attempted answers
C Questions
D Negative reactions

Figure 5-4. Bales interaction process analysis chart. (From Bales, R. [1950]. Interaction Process Analysis. Reading, MA: Addison Wesley, p. 59. Copyright 1950 by the University of Chicago.)

Member Role Observation

Leaders may also gather information from group observation by completing a member role form (Fig. 5-5). The members' names are placed at the top of the form, and a checkmark is placed in the column corresponding to the role that the member plays most often in the group. By filling out this form, leaders can quickly arrive at a rating of the different types of roles that were assumed by the participants in the group. This form also allows the observer to note any important roles that were not assumed by group members. If the leader–observer wants to record frequency of roles adopted, he or she can place a check in the column every time that the designated member has as-

MEMBER NAMES

ROLES									
TASK ROLES									
Initiator									
Information/Opinion Giver									
Information/Opinion Seeker									
Energizer									
Coordinator									
Recorder									
MAINTENANCE ROLES									
Encourager									
Harmonizer/Compromiser									
Gatekeeper									
Standard Setter									
Follower									
INDIVIDUAL ROLES									
Playboy									
Blocker									
Dominator									
Recognition Seeker									

Figure 5-5. Member role evaluation form.

sumed that particular role in the group. The various member roles are defined in Chapter 1.

Content and Process Analysis

An analysis of the content and process of a group session provides a basis for an evaluation of a group meeting. This procedure may be used by group leaders for their own analysis or by all group members for evaluation and discussion. The leader, member, or both should answer specific questions regarding content and process (Fig. 5-6), and a follow-up discussion should be focused on the ensuing information.

Analysis of Group Behavior

The leader can gain an understanding of group behavior by making observations of the nonverbal behavior of the members. Nonverbal communication, such as touching or gesturing while talking or listening, is frequently seen in a

---

Content Observations:

1. What were the main ideas presented in the discussion?
2. Which ideas were accepted?
3. Were there irrelevant ideas and discussion presented?
4. Did the group have the information necessary for making decisions?
5. Did the members talk about ideas and facts or feelings?

Process Observations:

1. Describe the tone of the discussion (e.g., friendly, tense, angry, anxious).
2. Is the atmosphere conducive to free expression? Why?
3. Identify any communication blocks (e.g., some members were not listened to; some were not understood; some were not recognized).
4. What factors seemed to keep the group from functioning well? (e.g., some members were uncomfortable; some couldn't hear because it was noisy; some seemed bored; and some came late. The group was not organized to do the job it was trying to do.)
5. What factors assisted the group's function?
6. Were there any indications of dissatisfaction with the kinds of decisions that were made by the group?

Figure 5-6. Content and process analysis.

group and can reveal how members feel about each other. Posture indicating inclusion or withdrawal is another form of nonverbal communication. For example, a member may lean toward the circle of members or away from them. Similarly, posture indicates interest and attention or boredom. If members of the group are sitting far apart from each other, this indicates that certain individuals feel isolated in the group. Eye contact and eye language may signal intimacy or confrontation, and avoidance of eye contact may mean reluctance to get involved. Sweeping eye contact often indicates a search for support or feedback.

Other types of member behavior can communicate meaning in the group. No behavior is random or accidental. Such things as eating, smoking, drinking, or visits to the bathroom can be gauges of the level of tension or boredom in the group. Periods of silence also have meanings. Observing how people look during periods of silence—sad, tense, contemplative—gives the leader clues about the members' feelings.

Meeting Evaluations

Leaders can ask members to evaluate meetings at the end of a session by completing evaluation forms. Howe (1968) reported the use of a brief rating form through which group members anonymously provide feedback in an occupational therapy activity group. On these forms, members checked whether they felt that the meeting was good, fair, or poor and whether they were able to express these feelings to the group. Knowles (1970) suggested an expanded evaluation form, which he calls an end-of-the-meeting form (Fig. 5-7). The design of this form allows members to make any comments they choose while also asking them to focus on the session just completed.

Date: Activity:
Please circle the phrase that best describes how you feel.

1. I think that in this meeting I learned
   a great deal   quite a lot   some   very little   nothing
2. On the whole, today's session was
   excellent   pretty good   all right   disappointing   terrible
3. I am leaving the meeting feeling
   enthusiastic   encouraged   all right   disappointed   frustrated
4. At this time, this activity interests me
   immensely   quite a bit   somewhat   a little   not at all

Comments: _____

_____

_____

Figure 5-7. Meeting evaluation form. (Adapted from Knowles, M. S. [1970]. The Modern Practice of Adult Education. New York: Association Press, p. 233.)

Coleadership

The use of coleaders in a group is recommended whenever possible, particularly for relatively inexperienced group leaders. Coleadership has several benefits. It is often difficult, even in a small group of six members, for the leader to attend to both the group process and the content at the same time. These tasks can be advantageously split up between the coleaders. For instance, the leader may be particularly attentive to what the group members are saying while the coleader may concentrate on the actions and reactions of the group members. Coleaders in a group may find opportunities to model interpersonal behaviors for group members. This can serve as an encouragement for members to explore new or tentative behaviors.

There are other advantages to a coleadership arrangement. Both leaders can contribute their observations to the preplanning process and to the postgroup evaluation. The planning and analysis will benefit from the dialogue.

Coleaders and other staff persons in a group need to be very sensitive to the amount of the groups' time they use. In an average group, which lasts 1 hour, there is less than 8 minutes per person of "air" time.

Conclusion

The leader of any group is responsible for assisting the group members to achieve their stated goals. Although the definition of a leader is still debated, research has developed several techniques that aid leaders in carrying out their roles. Not all of these strategies or techniques will be suitable for every leader and every group. Some leaders will be most comfortable using communication skills reinforced by the results of a sociogram; other leaders may find the evaluation forms especially valuable. Still, other leaders may find that the behavior of the group calls for modifications of these strategies. Each skill and each strategy must be adapted to suit the needs of the group.

Review Questions

1. What are the two categories of leadership functions? Do you need one or both to have a successful group? Are these functions the sole responsibility of the group leader?
2. What are the benefits gained from working with a coleader? Do any disadvantages exist?
3. If you have developed a good leadership style for working with groups of young children will this leadership style be equally good for a group of adults? What might need to be changed?
4. How can you gather the information necessary to help you design the leadership strategies you will need to use?

References

Bandura, A. (1969). Principles of Behavior Modification. New York: Holt Reinhart & Winston.

Bales, R. (1950). Interaction Process Analysis. Reading, MA: Addison Wesley.

Bradford, L., Stock, D., and Horwitz, M. (1978). How to diagnose group problems. In L. Bradford (ed.), Group Development (2nd ed.). La Jolla, CA: University Associates, pp. 62–78.

Egan, G. (1975). The Skilled Helper. Monterey, CA: Brooks/Cole.

Galigor, J. (1977). Perceptions of the group therapist and the dropout from group. In A. R. Wolberg and M. L. Aronson (eds.), Group Therapy 1977: An Overview. New York: Stratton Intercontinental Medical Book Corporation.

Homans, G. (1950). The Human Group. New York: Harcourt, Brace.

Hopkins, H., Smith, H., and Tiffany, E. G. (1983). Therapeutic application of activity. In H. Hopkins and H. Smith (eds.), Willard and Spackman's Occupational Therapy (6th ed.). Philadelphia: J. B. Lippincott.

Howe, M. C. (1968). An occupational therapy activity group. American Journal of Occupational Therapy 22(3): 176–179.

Johnson, D. W. (1972). Reaching Out: Interpersonal Effectiveness and Self-Actualization. Englewood Cliffs, NJ: Prentice-Hall.

Jourard, S. (1964). The Transparent Self. Princeton: Van Nostrand Company.

Knowles, M. S. (1970). The Modern Practice of Adult Education. New York: Association Press.

Lewin, K., Lippitt, R., and White, R. (1939). Patterns of aggressive behavior in experimentally created social climates. Journal of Social Psychology 10: 271–299.

Lieberman, M., Yalom, I., and Miles, M. (1973). Encounter Groups: First Facts. New York: Basic Books.

Lippitt, G. L. (1961). How to get results from a group. In L. P. Bradford (ed.), Group Development. La Jolla, CA: University Associates, pp. 31–36.

Napier, N., and Gershenfeld, M. (1973). Groups: Theory and Experience. Boston: Houghton Mifflin.

Rogers, C. (1959). Theory of therapy-personality and interpersonal relationships. In S. Koch (ed.), Psychology: A Study of a Science (vol. 3). New York: McGraw-Hill.

Rogers, C. (1967). The process of the basic encounter group. In J. Bugental (ed.), Challenges of Humanistic Psychology. New York: McGraw-Hill, p. 270.

Schwartzberg, S., Howe, M., and McDermott, A. (1982). A comparison of three treatment group formats for facilitating social interaction. Occupational Therapy in Mental Health: A Journal for Psychosocial Practice and Research 2(4): 1–16.

Stogdill, R. M. (1948). Personality factors associated with leadership: A survey of the literature. Journal of Psychology 25: 3–71.

Tannenbaum, R., and Schmidt, W. H. (1958). How to choose a leadership pattern. Harvard Business Review 36 (March–April): 95–101.

Yalom, I. (1970). The Theory and Practice of Group Psychotherapy. New York: Basic Books.

Chapter **6**
Stage One: Design

The functional group is a procedure directed toward the use of time and energy in purposeful action in order to promote adaptation through occupation. Such groups progress through four successive, interdependent stages. These stages are design, formation, development, and termination.

Unlike the other stages, stage one involves only the group leader or coleaders and covers the leader's preparation prior to actual group formation and implementation (Box 6-1). Although issues related to the other three stages may first arise in the design stage, those issues are not resolved at this point. The main purpose of the design stage is to establish the initial group structure for the next stage: the formation stage.

The specific leader functions of this stage are as follows:

- Assessing the need for a group
- Determining group goals and methods
- Developing a group plan
- Selecting group members
- Structuring the group and its tasks

Beginning with this chapter, we shall follow three groups through the successive stages. These three groups are identified as Open Occupational Therapy Group: Case Study Number 1, Closed Occupational Therapy Group: Case Study Number 2, and Community-Based Occupational Therapy Group: Case Study Number 3. The first two case studies are groups meeting within a clinical or hospital environment. The third group is part of a program held in a community center for senior citizens. In addition to the standard forms useful to the leader in this stage, we have included completed sample forms for the case studies.

Assessing Need and Support

The functional group is aimed at individuals who have experienced a physical injury or illness; suffer from an emotional, developmental, social, or congenital disorder; or have difficulty in dealing with the aging process and need assistance in adapting to their life situations (Box 6-2). Sometimes, in community-based groups the goals are to maintain wellness. To eliminate any confusion about the focus of this group in light of the wide range of possible members, we shall further clarify the purpose of the group by stating what it is not. The functional group is *not*:

Box 6-1
Stage One

The purpose of this chapter is to describe the leadership tasks of the design stage.

- Restricted to particular settings, such as inpatient or outpatient settings
- Aimed at treating the etiology of diseases
- Aimed at teaching components of skills in isolation
- Aimed at teaching isolated behaviors
- Product-oriented as the goal is not a product alone
- Focused solely on primary process, on developing insight, and delving into psychohistorical issues
- Aimed at teaching a progression of age/stage-specific skills or behaviors
- Aimed primarily at rendering a cost-effective service

The specific types of approaches just excluded are the domain of other models; for instance, psychoanalytic groups are better prepared to delve into historical issues. The functional group focuses on aiding an individual's adaptation through purposeful, self-initiated, spontaneous, and group centered activity.

To determine the suitability of a group membership for any individual, the leader usually conducts an initial needs assessment. The functional group would be an appropriate tool for an individual with the following needs:

- Evaluating occupational behaviors necessary for functioning in life roles
- Achieving the occupational behaviors prerequisite to successful functioning in life roles
- Preventing deterioration of occupational behaviors necessary for adaptation
- Facilitating the maintenance of health or state of adaptation

The needs listed here are broader than those listed in the categories of excluded needs. They also include needs of groups as social systems. The emphasis is on quality of functioning in a community rather than on mastery of a given skill or resolution of a specific problem. In community-based groups, the goals of a group may be based on the needs identified by the clients rather than the needs addressed by the occupational therapist. In this case, the needs assessment section of the standard form presented at the end of this chapter may be omitted or altered. Encouraging members to identify their own needs for the group, whenever they can, serves to increase their direct participation in activities.

Occupational therapists see patients at various points in the continuum of care. Depending on the problem, the therapist may meet the prospective group member in a peer support group; an acute care section of a general hospital; a spinal cord injury unit; rehabilitation hospital; a nursing home; an outpatient facility, such as a school, day program, or partial hospitalization program that provides transitional or long-term care; or in a family or care-giver group in the community (Box 6-3). Prospective group members may have a variety of disorders, such as head injury, schizophrenia, borderline personality disorder, mental illness, cerebrovascular accident, fracture, burn, spinal cord injury, arthritis, or Alzheimer's disease or may be in need of support or preventive health services. The members may also be of varying ages—from a child to an older adult—and may be from a variety of socioeconomic backgrounds and educational or functional levels.

The diversity of setting and population with which occupational therapists work offers a variety of opportunities for initiating functional groups. Nevertheless, the decision to offer a functional group depends in part on an institution's aims and the roles and functions of the institution's health professionals. The professionals who deliver the services are typically not the same people who decide on the programs to be offered. In addition, member needs may not be the most significant factor in a decision. In discussing inpatient group psychotherapy, Yalom (1983) points out, "Decisions about number, types, and frequency of groups are often made on the basis of what will not ruffle the staff rather than of what will be most effective for the patient" (p. 15). Funding also can play a role in determining the types of services offered. For many reasons, occupational therapists rarely seek to work without a connection to an institutional setting—clinical or community. Even therapists who conduct functional groups on a private practice basis usually work in collaboration with a referring physician or agency. Self-advocacy and family-centered models of care appear to have a growing influence on the types of groups offered.

Because of their dependence on institutions, payers, and referring parties, occupational therapists must educate other professionals and nonprofessionals within these settings on the value of functional groups (Box 6-4). When an occupational therapist identifies a community of individuals who might benefit from a functional group, the therapist could present the initial needs assessment and expected outcomes to persuade those responsible for a final decision to consider offering such a program (Box 6-5). This is when data from outcome studies or research done in similar groups becomes extremely helpful. Thera-

---

Box 6-3
Flexible, Adaptive

Because of the broad nature of its goals, the functional group can be held in a variety of clinical and nonclinical settings.

Box 6-4
Spreading the Word

The realities of today's health care environment necessitate that occupational therapists educate other professionals and nonprofessionals about the values and benefits of functional groups.

Box 6-5
Supportive Resources

Some considerations to keep in mind about available resources are:

- The people supporting you in the community or institution
- Streams of funding that are readily available
- Additional funding and resources that you need to seek out
- Data-based information to back up the efficacy and postulated outcomes of the group plan

pists can profitably take some time to accumulate this kind of outcome data regarding the groups they lead. Even the outcome data from a few small groups can be convincing (Box 6-6).

Screening mechanisms should be tailored to individual settings and populations. Therapists must determine if individuals need assistance in maintaining or developing occupational behaviors to function effectively in their life roles. They must also determine if a health maintenance program is needed within the institution. Specific methods of assessment have been devised and can be found in the occupational therapy literature (Barris, Kielhofner, and Watts, 1983; Hemphill, 1982; Mosey, 1973). In examining evaluation data, the therapist should ask several questions. Are there individuals who need help to effectively carry out and maintain their roles? Does this institution have a structure for maintaining health? Will this institution support the aims of a functional group? Finally, occupational therapists working in the well community must address one additional question: Does this environment maintain health and prevent deterioration of occupational behaviors necessary for human adaptation?

Determining Group Goals and Methods

After the leader has determined the need for a functional group, he or she must determine group goals and methods (Box 6-7). The leader can determine the prospective member's goals through one of three techniques: pregroup inter-

Box 6-6
Needs Assessment and Documentation

The ongoing process for goal-setting and documentation is usually accomplished with the group members. To help guide this process, the following questions can be asked to determine the best way to proceed:

1. Even though a client in a community-based program may enroll in a group without a medical referral indicating the goals for participation, is it still important to make a needs assessment?

2. Who should make the needs assessment and/or set the goals for the group:
   a. the client,
   b. the occupational therapist,
   c. the group, or
   d. all the above?

3. Does there also need to be an evaluation process to:
   a. document the program's efficacy for the sponsoring agency,
   b. document the progress, or lack of progress of the clients,
   c. help guide the leader in structuring the group sessions,
   d. determine the clients' satisfaction,
   e. document the client's progress in the event of litigation, or
   f. document the program for purposes of reimbursement?

4. If you lead a group for six weeks and then terminate that group and start a new series of groups for another six weeks, do you need to make an assessment and evaluation for each series of groups? Why?

5. If you have no control over attendance, the referral process, or reimbursement, is this a therapy group or a support group? What are the legal and ethical implications regarding your responsibility to the group members and agency?

6. What would you like to know about this group after the initial meetings, midpoint, and at the termination of the group?
   a. How would you gather this information?
   b. Of what importance would this information be to you, to your financial supporters, and to your sponsors?
   c. Do you see a need for keeping records of individual change as well as the group's process?

view, group history, or member assessment. Each technique is best suited to a particular circumstance; for example, the group history is designed for an institution that has an existing group that will be changed to a functional group. If the leader chooses to have the group members contribute to establishing the group goals, the leader may set tentative goals for the first meeting until members have an opportunity to state their own needs and goals.

> Box 6-7
> **Key to Success**
>
> For a group to be successful, group members should perceive the group as congruent with their needs and goals.

Pregroup Interview

The pregroup interview technique is designed to elicit the goals of prospective group members, as well as to provide general information about the members. The leader can achieve several purposes with this interview: establish the member's level of functioning in occupational behaviors, self-perceived needs, and functional goals; form a beginning therapeutic rapport with the member; and explain the nature, expectations, and general purposes of a functional group. If someone else is doing the pregroup interview, as sometimes happens in a community-based group, the occupational therapists should outline the information that he or she needs from the prospective members and also the information that needs to be communicated to them.

On the basis of initial interviews, the group leader tentatively outlines the group's general goals and methods before the initial meeting. This plan represents the starting point for the group and should be modified in an ongoing fashion as the group becomes a more cohesive unit. Ultimately, goal setting and program planning should be a collaborative process between group leaders and members as the group moves through successive stages.

Group History

If an established group exists, the leader can take a group history. This history should include answers to the questions shown on the Group History Form in Display 6-1. The group history is usually constructed from the group's records rather than from interviewing members. Including a clear statement of former and current goals of both individuals and the group as a whole is important. The group history can be used in conjunction with the third technique, assessment of members. In some instances, the group members or relatives may interview the group leader and together construct the history and goals. This method is particularly important when the leader is in the role of consultant or facilitator.

Member Assessment

If the occupational therapist has identified prospective members in a setting that allows the therapist to evaluate the individual's abilities in a wide range of areas, the therapist may use a member assessment such as the one shown in

---

Display 6-1   Group History Form

Name of Group _____

Date_____

1. How long has the group been in existence? What is its anticipated duration? What is its general stage and level of development? Who has authority over goals and structure of the group?

2. How was the group leadership and membership determined (voluntary or involuntary, and so on)?

3. How stable is the group membership? What is the rate of attendance? Is it an open or closed group? If it is an open group, are there any new members in the group? How long have the new and old members been in the group? What outcomes have been achieved by the group and individuals? In what ways has the group or leadership been unsuccessful? If it is a closed group, what criteria are used to select the members? How often and for how long a time did the group meet?

4. What is the existing group structure? Who has ultimate authority to change this structure?

5. What other factors, from the group's history, are pertinent to your understanding, assessing, and planning for the group (such as prior group leadership style)?

Howe, M., & Schwartzberg, S. (2001). A Functional Approach to Group Work in Occupational Therapy (3rd ed.).

Display 6-2. For example, a therapist in an inpatient institution could use this technique, but the leader of an open group in a setting outside a medical care institution would probably not. The assessment of members suggested here covers all facets of the member's health (diagnosis and treatment) and behavior (cognitive, psychosocial, neuromotor, and physical), as well as the member's general and specific goals. If possible, the leader or therapist should include an assessment of the member's performance and achievements to date.

In addition to the three techniques for collecting information on the possible goals of the group, the leader should consider the setting of the group and determine if the setting will influence the group's goals. The assessment should include the physical location, emotional environment, and administrative structure of the institution containing or sponsoring the group (see Display 6-2).

Display 6-2   Assessment of Members Form
---

1. Assessment of Group Members (Including Range of Behaviors)
   A. General description (include significant demographic and medical/psychological information)

   B. General description of members' expected environment (include specific information regarding where and with whom the group members will live and reside, as well as expected roles)

   C. Description of current performance in areas of occupational behavior
   Work:

   Self-care:

   Leisure:

   D. Cognitive behavior

   E. Psychosocial behavior

   F. Physical and neuromotor behavior

   G. What is the significance of these factors with regard to individual member goals and forming or planning the group or group session(s)?

2. Assessment of Group Context (the Facility)
   A. General description of program in which group is included (administrative structure)

   B. General description of physical environment

continued

Display 6-2   Assessment of Members Form (*Continued*)

C. General description of emotional climate

D. Frame of reference, purpose, and objectives

E. What is the significance of these factors in forming or planning the group or group session(s)?

3. Assessment of Environmental Supports and Constraints
   A. Facilities and materials

   B. Scheduling

   C. Group norms and prior therapy group experience (if any)

   D. Do any of the environmental constraints require modification of the group, or could you alter the situation (such as locating needed materials)?

Howe, M., & Schwartzberg, S. (2001). A Functional Approach to Group Work in Occupational Therapy (3rd ed.).

After the therapist has collected information concerning the members and their goals, he or she can distill from the many general and specific goals a set of goals that relate to all group members. For clarity, the goals should be stated in behavioral terms with desired outcome criteria although the functional group does not have a behavioral frame of reference. The leader should state the general behavioral goals for the client group (behaviors that are to be increased or decreased). Because setting goals is a continuing process usually done in conjunction with the members, the leader's initial goals may change over time (Box 6-8). The therapist should also state, in behavioral terms, the criteria for successful attainment of goals in each session. As Yalom (1983) has clearly stated, "Appropriate goal setting is of crucial importance to the proper functioning of the small therapy group. Overly ambitious goals impair the effectiveness of the group and lower the morale of the therapist" (p. 62).

Depending on the goals, the therapist should select a methodology. This might include activities such as participating in structured exercises or identifying the activity for the group. The methodology should suit the group's gen-

Box 6-8
Assessment Data

The assessment of members of a functional group should include:

- Health
- Behavior
- Member goals
- Member performance and achievements

eral goals, time frame, and structure. Just as group goals, methods should be regularly adjusted to the pace of the group and its development.

Developing a Group Plan

After the leader establishes general goals and methods, he or she should develop a general group plan, which provides the leader with a tentative structure or cognitive strategy for interactions with the group. The plan also serves as a guide for program planning while keeping the group working toward its goals. The strategies, it should be emphasized, change as leaders interact with the group and reflect on their observations. Nevertheless, in all circumstances, the leader needs a specific format; this is especially true for open groups and acute care settings. In these circumstances, the leader might have only one contact with a group member; consequently, each session must have optimal impact.

In addition to a general group plan for the overall group structure (Box 6-9), the therapist should develop a group session plan for each session. A session evaluation form is used to review the group's progress and aid in reformulating the group session plan.

General Group Plan

The general group plan sets forth the overall framework for the group, from formation through termination. The plan presents a detailed statement of goals;

Box 6-9
Sharing the Plan

The general group plan should be made available to all staff involved in the care of a group member.

criteria for achieving the goals; criteria for selecting group members, leadership roles, and functions; requirements for group members; and selected group methods and procedures, techniques, and strategies (see the General Group Plan Protocol in Display 6-3). The goals presented are long-term and represent what should be achieved at the group's termination (closed group) or at an individual member's departure from the group (open group). The methods listed are procedural guides for planning and implementing specific techniques and modalities for achieving group goals. Because of its detail, the general plan is usually based on a group history or assessment of members. If these methods of assessment are not possible, initial group sessions may focus on member assessment and evaluation to develop a detailed plan. When a group is being organized for the first time, the general plan will probably have to be formulated following the first meeting of the group when the pertinent information becomes available.

Group Session Plan

The group session plan establishes the specific framework for one session (or unit of sessions) designed to partially fulfill a specific aspect of the general group plan. Goals are short-term and indicate the anticipated group achievement for the specific session or unit. The session plan also includes specific techniques and modalities for the session or unit (see Display 6-4).

Session Evaluation Form

As the group moves through its periods of development, the leader should evaluate the progress of the group and its members. A sample session evaluation form is presented in Display 6-5 to assist the leader in evaluating the group's progress toward long-term and short-term goals. The leader may also gather information on whether or not the selected techniques and modalities are appropriate for the group and on the effect of his or her own leadership behavior on the group. Changes are made according to the evaluations. The data collected can also be used to modify the general group plan and, later, group session plans.

Selecting Group Members

The functional group is open to anyone who has a physical injury or illness; has an emotional, developmental, or congenital disorder; or has difficulty coping with the aging process or changes in the environment. This description includes the elderly and adolescents. The group is also open to individuals who need a structure to maintain adaptation or to prevent deterioration of occupational behavior and adaptive skills. Membership may also include individuals who wish to change the structure of a natural group such as a family or work group.

Despite the broad description of individuals suitable for the functional group, not everyone can benefit from this format. According to Yalom (1983):

Display 6-3   General Group Plan Proto

A. Name of Group

B. Time/length of meeting(s)

C. Place

D. Open or closed group
   Statement of rationale:

E. Group goals:

   Depending on the specific group, these may include primary and secondary objectives and leader objectives for group as a whole and/or individual members.
   1. Goals (behaviors you wish to increase or decrease)

   2. Rationale for goal selection

   3. Outcome criteria for successful goal attainment in session(s) stated in behavioral terms

F. Group composition or criteria for selecting members

G. Leadership roles and functions

H. Characteristics of group contract

I. Group methods and procedures to be employed: Briefly describe or list methods, techniques, and modalities

---

Howe, M., & Schwartzberg, S. (2001). A Functional Approach to Group Work in Occupational Therapy (3rd ed.).

Display 6-4   Group Session Plan Protocol

A. Name of Group _____

   Date_____

B. Specific goals for the group session

C. Specific goals for group members if different from those mentioned already and goals for each group member

D. Description of and rationale for methods and procedures

E. Description of and rationale for leadership role

F. Describe necessary preparations

G. List material and equipment needed

H. Time and sequence outline for sessions, including what you will do and say as leader and what the group will do; consider both content and process

I. Other information pertinent to this specific session: For example: Will there be any new members, coleaders, or guests? Is there an unusual tone on the unit or special event that is about to occur or just occurred for the individual member or group?

Howe, M., & Schwartzberg, S. (2001). A Functional Approach to Group Work in Occupational Therapy (3rd ed.).

There is considerable consensus in the research literature that psychotic patients are most successfully treated in supportive, reality-focused, structured group therapy and require a sealing over rather than an opening up. . . . They are made more anxious by an unstructured group experience and do less well in groups if they disclose a great deal about themselves. . . . An extensive review of the entire clinical literature reaches the same conclusions: psychotic patients do far better in inpatient therapy groups that are reality- or activity-oriented rather than in insight-oriented ones. . . . A review of group therapy in day treatment centers yields the identical conclusion: group therapy aimed at insight and derepression is contraindicated for the schizophrenic patient. (p. 32)

Display 6-5   Session Evaluation Form Protocol

A. Name of Group _____

   Date_____

B. Were the goals accomplished? (Give rationale and state outcome).

   Was the session helpful in accomplishing short- and long-term group and individual member goals?

   Do you have any evidence that the session(s) have been helpful to the members' functioning (adaptation) outside of the group?

C. Was the group structure adequate for accomplishing the goals? Give rationale, and consider: leadership; time/length of meeting; open versus closed group; time, sequence, methods and procedures; media/modalities/techniques employed; norms/behaviors reinforced implicitly or explicitly; methods of reinforcement; and stage of group's development.

   Did the structure provide optimal "action" or "flow activity" for a "flow state" to occur?

   Did the structure provide optimal purposeful, self-initiated, spontaneous, and group-centered "action" for cognitive and emotional impact, skill learning, and adaptation to occur through "occupation"?

   Did the structure provide for new learning or reinforcement of current level of functioning or adaptation, or did it reinforce functioning below current level of adaptation? Explain and give rationale.

   Did the structure provide an opportunity for evaluation and feedback regarding the group procedures and member progress? Explain.

D. What changes would you make regarding group goals and structure for the next session, or if you were to lead this session again?

E. Were you adequately prepared for the session? (Give rationale, considering such things as time, place, materials, and physical and emotional environment.)

F. How did you function as leader? How did your behavior and role affect the group? Were you effective? (Give rationale.) What did you learn about yourself as group leader?

continued

Display 6-5   Session Evaluation Form Protocol (*Continued*)

G. Was the group interaction as you anticipated? If problems occurred, what processes can you identify as a basis for understanding the problems?

H. In the future, what might you do differently as group leader? (Give rationale.)

Howe, M., & Schwartzberg, S. (2001). A Functional Approach to Group Work in Occupational Therapy (3rd ed.).

Depending on the nature of the particular group, psychotic patients need not necessarily be excluded. The group can be oriented so that it is highly supportive. Further, the aim of the functional group is not insight or the examination of unconscious material alone. Indeed, the functional group is clearly reality-oriented.

Because peer groups play an important part in the normal development of adolescents, the functional group is particularly well suited to this age group. Adolescents need strong peer support to feel adequate. They are also developing a sense of self or personal identity and competency through testing a variety of behaviors. The activity and action orientation of the functional group match the modes of expression most often used by adolescents to explore their questions of identity and growth.

The wide range of individuals who are suited to the functional group indicates that the essential criteria qualifying an individual for the group are broad. There are five general criteria for the group member. Each member should be able to do the following:

- Communicate verbally, in a simple manner.
- Understand simple communications, such as instructions (written or verbal).
- Be able to focus on a structured task in the presence of two other group members for a minimum of 30 minutes. This time may be different for children or others where group is planned with short attention span in mind.
- Understand the purpose and nature of the group and the roles of the members and leader.
- Tolerate the stimulation of interpersonal contact.

After considering an individual's general qualifications for membership, the leader must consider other factors. The group must be formed so that members work together in reasonable order. The number of possible members is therefore limited, as is the range of problems and goals that can be dealt with. In forming a particular group, the therapist must next consider composition and size.

Group Composition

A leader can determine the composition of a group according to one of three techniques. First, the leader can select members who are alike, who have similar adaptation problems or needs. The leader can look for similarity in skill deficit, role disorder, developmental disability, illness or injury, diagnosis, or age. Second, the leader can select members who have the same type of adaptation problem but in varying degrees. Third, the leader can select members who have a variety of adaptation problems. Regardless of the criteria of composition, the leader should compose the group so that it will be a cohesive one.

No methods can guarantee a cohesive group. According to Yalom (1970), "There appears to be a general clinical sentiment that heterogeneous groups have advantages over homogeneous groups for intensive interactional group therapy" (p. 193). He continues, "Although group cohesiveness is by no means synonymous with therapy outcome, there is considerable evidence ... that cohesiveness is positively related to outcome and may be considered a way station or an intervening variable" (pp. 197–198).

In composing a group, the leader selects members who have similar goals, abilities, and needs and who can function together in a particular action or activity (Box 6-10). It is unlikely, therefore, that a recently admitted patient with a cerebrovascular accident would be assigned to a group with patients who are preparing for immediate discharge. The treatment goals and functional abilities would be too diverse. By contrast, two patients preparing for the home-maker role, one with an upper extremity fracture and one with joint inflammation from arthritis, might be quite compatible members of the same group. Again, the goals of the group and the treatment modality or activity process need to be considered when members are chosen for a specific group.

Group Size

The size of a group will influence how the members relate to each other and other facets of the group experience. No strict rule dictates size. According to Yalom (1970), five to ten members is an acceptable number for an "interactional therapy group." He considers approximately seven members ideal (p. 215). We agree with this figure; seven members can work together effectively in the activity of the group and participate fully in the process of the group. Yalom (1970) also points out that if a group has fewer than five members, the opportunity for maximal member interaction decreases and the therapy becomes more leader centered. When the group size increases beyond ten members, there is less time for individual members. In our practice we found that size should be based in part on members' attention spans, functional abilities, and ability to delay grat-

---

Box 6-10
Cohesion Valued

Functional group leaders are not required to compose heterogeneous groups, but they should attempt to create cohesive ones.

ification. If members have problems in these areas, groups for these individuals should have fewer than five members. Again following Yalom (1970), leaders should compose a group with two more members than the ideal size. One or two members will drop out at the beginning, and the two additional members will ensure that overall size does not fall below the minimum needed. Leaders should also consider special problems related to settings. In acute care settings, patient turnover is high, and rapid discharge is common. The size of the group should be large enough to absorb sudden changes in membership.

Structuring the Group and Tasks

The functional group uses occupational performance (purposeful action) to achieve treatment goals. To do this, the group should be structured to accomplish specific aspects of working in a group that will in turn lead to the ultimate goal. The group should be designed to achieve the following:

- Maximal involvement of members through group-centered action
- Maximal sense of individual and group identity
- A "flow experience"
- Spontaneous involvement
- Member support and feedback

As Yalom (1983) points out, "Group leaders provide structure for the group by delineating clear spatial and temporal boundaries; by adopting a lucid, decisive, but flexible personal style; by providing an explicit orientation and preparation for the patient; and by developing a consistent, coherent group procedure" (p. 108).

Maximal Involvement

Maximal involvement is achieved through four steps. The leader must make each step clear and set the pace for the members.

Step One: Orient the Group to the Design
The leader should first explain the nature of the group and purpose of the session(s). The leader and member roles, as well as specific goals, should be made explicit in the leader's introductory remarks to the group. The group's format or structure should make sense in terms of the group members' specific needs and perceptions.

Step Two: Explain Procedures to Group
After the orientation, the leader should explain the procedure(s) to be used in the session(s). The group methodology, specific tasks, sequence of activities, agenda, and purpose must be stated in an unambiguous manner.

Step Three: Set Up the Task
Depending on the nature of the group and the abilities of the members, the leader may involve the group in setting up the task or may do this for the group. The group may also be involved in the clean-up period after the activity has ended.

Step Four: Follow-Up

After the group participates in the task, the leader assists the group in assessing the experience. The leader guides the group in connecting the task experience to the group goals and individual member goals.

Maximal Sense of Individual and Group Identity

The therapist must create a climate of safety within the group through support and genuine caring. The tasks should be structured so members feel in control of the process. This is accomplished by involving the members in setting goals, selecting and implementing tasks, and doing follow-up. The therapist designs these experiences at the level of the members' abilities. An open group may require the therapist to highly structure these procedures.

Flow Experience

In structuring a flow experience, the leader attempts to create opportunities or challenges for action. This involves creating an environment that stimulates curiosity and the desire to achieve. Csikszentmihalyi (1975) describes a "model of the flow state," which should serve as a guideline for the therapist. He states:

> When a person believes that his action opportunities are too demanding for his capabilities, the resulting stress is experienced as anxiety; when the ratio of capabilities is higher, but the challenges are still too demanding for his skills, the experience is worry. The state of flow is felt when opportunities for action are in balance with the actor's skills; the experience is then autotelic. When skills are greater than opportunities for using them, the state of boredom results; this state again fades into anxiety when the ratio becomes too large. (p. 49)

In designing a task that will enable the members to achieve a "flow experience," the leader should include only those tasks that are culturally acceptable to the members and that can produce personal satisfaction. Simultaneously, the leader can find that a member's flow experience in an activity group may also be frustrating at times. In his study of play and flow in an activity group, Persson (1996) believes that, in spite of cultural expectations, adult participants dropped the achievement demands in favor of nonverbal expression such as painting. He explains that, "paradoxically, the np/nf [non-play/non-flow] state,

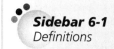

Sidebar 6-1
Definitions

Functional group: *A procedure in which time and energy are used in purposeful action in order to promote adaptation through occupation*

Flow state: *An experience in which opportunities for action are in balance with the individual's skills*

as it generally preceded the development of p/f [play/flow], could be interpreted as a prerequisite for p/f " (p. 40).

Spontaneous Involvement

The leader must guide the group toward discussion and action in the present; this is achieved through modeling behaviors and feedback. In addition, the activities should be structured so that action is required. The leader in turn relates the group's and individual member's behavior to the purpose of the session(s) (Fig. 6-1).

Support and Feedback

During a session, the leader should demonstrate specific modes of support to encourage members in their participation. The leader should follow these basic principles.

- The leader points out universal elements, needs, concerns, and reactions to group members.
- Members are never criticized, blamed, or made to feel isolated.
- The activities are structured according to the range of members' abilities.
- The leader is empathetic and teaches members how to give feedback constructively.

Specific skills, such as empathy and genuineness, modeling behavior, giving feedback, and reality testing, are discussed in detail in Chapter 5.

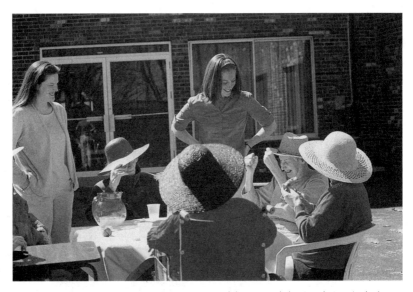

Figure 6-1. Spontaneous group action. (Photograph by Sarah Brezinsky.)

Leader Emotional Response

The design stage may elicit mixed feelings for the group leader. In starting a new venture, feelings of anxiety and excitement related to the challenges ahead may surface. Feelings surface whether the group is preformed or newly created. If a group is preformed, someone other than the group leader selected the members. This may be an administrator or clinical supervisor. In such an instance, the leader may be concerned about whether there is a good match between his or her skills and members' needs. Feelings of insecurity may arise if the existing group had a positive attachment to the prior leader. Likewise, if the previous leader had negative or resistive relationships, there may be concern. In this instance, the leader may even experience extreme feelings, such as panic. This is especially true when leaders expect to rescue the group or have fantasies of saving the members. If the group is a newly created one, the leader may be fraught with anxieties concerning whether there will be enough members, sufficient reimbursement, and adequate means to market the program. The area of highest anxiety in starting a new group is often the leader's fear of "getting off on the wrong foot." In planning the group's initial sessions, the leader may need reassurance that it is natural not to find total group participation; "maximal involvement" is a more realistic goal.

The group's history (see Group History, Display 6-1, Case Studies 1, 2, and 3 Group History) can help leaders self-examine their emotional responses and to identify patterns in their own reactions to working in the design stage. Self-reflective questions can aid this analysis (Box 6-11).

Box 6-11
Leader Questions

The leader asks the following self-reflective questions in the design stage:

- Will the plan be effective? What are my concerns about my own competence? Are these concerns realistic? Who can help me assess my strengths and areas for growth? What learning resources are available such as an academic advisor or supervisor?

- Will there be a sufficient number of members? What are my concerns about acceptance and reasons for working with this group? Am I being realistic? Where can I get my emotional, social, and spiritual needs met outside of the group setting?

- Will there be attrition and will I get paid? What are my concerns about loss? Are they realistic concerns? Who can be a resource to help me sort this out?

Conclusion

The leader role in the design stage is of critical importance to the group's ultimate success. In this stage, the leader must assess the need for a group, determine group goals and methods, develop a plan, select group members, and structure the group and its tasks. In developing a group plan, the leader aims to create a structure for facilitating purposeful, self-initiated, spontaneous, and group-centered action. Although a carefully monitored group structure has been emphasized in this chapter, one should also bear in mind that contingency or alternate plans may be necessitated. The initial plans are preliminary. The group format may need adaptations when the group begins its sessions or as it proceeds through its various stages of development. To illustrate the principles and concerns of the design stage, we have included general group plan protocols for the two groups described in the case studies.

CASE STUDY NUMBER 1
Open Occupational Therapy Group

Group History

1. This group has existed on the psychiatric inpatient unit for 3 years. It is expected to continue as a part of the unit's occupational therapy program. This is an open group, with the membership changing on a weekly, often daily, basis. Because the membership changes, the group is always, in a sense, in the design stage, as well as proceeding through all the functional group stages. The chief of psychiatric services, a psychiatrist, has ultimate authority over the goals and structure of any therapies conducted on the unit. The occupational therapists have direct responsibility for designing, implementing, and evaluating the groups they conduct.

2. The occupational therapists—or for our purposes, the functional group leaders—established the criteria for group membership. After assessing the needs of the hospital's psychiatric inpatient population, the leaders, in consultation with the staff, determined that at any given time there would be eight patients in need of such a group. Because the inpatient unit is an acute, voluntary, open psychiatric service, the group, herein named the Project Group, has voluntary membership.

3. The group meets daily for 45 minutes. It is an open group, and daily attendance is required. Usually, new members enter and depart from the group on a daily basis.

4. In addition to the Project Group, patients attend daily community meetings, group psychotherapy, individual counseling, and occupational therapy sessions. Most members are also being treated with psychotropic medications or are being evaluated for such treatment. Each patient has

his or her own case manager. All treatment is supervised by the patient's attending psychiatrist.

5. Some of the patients are readmissions and have attended the Project Group in prior hospitalizations. Other patients have no group treatment experience or have had psychosocial treatment in other settings.

Assessment of Members

1. Assessment of Group Members (Including Range of Behaviors)

   A. General description
   Patients primarily live in the communities surrounding the hospital area. The group is conducted on the psychiatric inpatient unit of an urban private general hospital. The unit has 16 beds and an interdisciplinary staff consisting of mental health counselors, nurses, occupational therapists, psychiatrists, psychologists, and social workers. Most patients are middle-class to upper middle-class blue-collar and white-collar workers. All hospitalization costs are being covered through third-party payers. Diagnoses include affective disorders, schizophrenic disorders, personality disorders, substance use disorders, and eating disorders. Some patients have medical problems, such as cardiac conditions, arthritis, diabetes, and multiple sclerosis, but these conditions are stabilized and secondary to the psychiatric disorder. All patients are between 16 and 70 years of age.

   B. General description of members' expected environment
   All group members are expected to return to their homes in the commu nity or to find a more suitable living arrangement in the community. Members are parents, workers, students, or retirees.

   C. Description of current performance in areas of occupational behavior
   Work: Two members are college freshmen, three are homemakers, one is retired, and two are employed (an accountant and a freelance writer). Self-care: All are independent in basic self-care; they have difficulty making decisions when human transactions are involved in their self-care or care of their environment.
   Leisure: All members have expressed dissatisfaction with their use of leisure time. Some feel they have few to no interests; are all either consumed with work or do not have the resources (people, places, money, and so forth) to participate in nonvocational activities.

   D. Cognitive behavior
   Members are able to understand simple written and verbal instructions, and can concentrate on a structured task minimally for 30 minutes and maximally for 45 minutes. All have intact memory skills. Members are well oriented to time, place, and person. The majority of members have some insight into current difficulties. Some members have difficulty sequencing a plan of action when solving problems, whereas others are

able to make abstract judgments but have difficulty with simple decisions involved in daily living.

E. Psychosocial behavior

Members have difficulty recognizing and verbalizing their emotions. Although members are able to imitate behaviors, they have difficulty identifying when a change in action is needed. Some members rely totally on others to fulfill their needs, whereas others are unwilling to accept suggestions or help. Most members are unable to identify their strengths and therefore focus their discussions on limitations. Several members are unable to handle frustration with a task and show anxiety by not completing the activity, moving about restlessly, or being irritable while attempting to complete the task. Members attempt to interact with others in a group by always offering help (often to the exclusion of asking for help), by demanding assistance and withdrawing if it is not immediately available, or by vacillating between these extremes.

F. Physical and neuromotor behavior

All members are ambulatory and all have adequate gross and fine coordination and range of motion to perform routine activities of daily living. They are all able to maintain balance when performing table activities, walking, and running. Many are unable to perform tasks with the strength and endurance required for the members' prehospitalization routines; for example, they may take frequent rests, or complain of strain or fatigue.

G. What is the significance of these factors with regard to individual member goals and forming or planning the group or group session(s)?

To promote total participation, ideally the group should be composed of no more than eight members (men and women) and have two leaders (one male and one female). The group will need to be advised on how to select relatively short-term activities with little complexity and opportunity for error. The leaders will need to assume an active role in adapting the activities so that a variety of group membership roles can be practiced. They will also need to observe the group's process, suggest alternative behaviors, and assume group membership and leadership roles when the members are unable to do so. A highly supportive, genuine, and consistent emotional climate must be established and reinforced by the leaders.

2. **Assessment of Group Context (the Facility)**

   A. General description of program in which group is included (administrative structure)

   The group is part of the milieu therapy program offered to patients on the psychiatric inpatient unit. It is a service provided by the hospital's staff occupational therapists working on the unit. The inpatient unit is one of the services offered through the hospital's department of psychiatry.

B. General description of physical environment

The unit has a long hallway with eight semiprivate rooms, with a kitchen at one end, and the nurses' station, occupational therapy room, staff offices, and community living room at the other end. The occupational therapy room has one long rectangular table, a small circular table, work benches, and activity supply cabinets along the walls. The room is painted in soft beige; patients' projects are scattered about; and there are many hanging plants over a large work sink.

C. General description of emotional climate

The emotional climate varies according to the patient population on the unit. At times, the atmosphere appears calm and quiet, and at other times it is noisy, high-keyed, and energetic.

D. Frame of reference, purpose, and objectives

Using a biopsychosocial model, this short-term unit provides a safe environment for patients who have demonstrated self-destructive behaviors. Its primary purposes are evaluation, alleviation of acute symptoms of the patient's psychiatric condition, and referral to outpatient services in the community.

E. What is the significance of these factors for forming or planning the group or group session(s)?

Because of the high patient turnover, the sessions must be held and planned on a daily basis. Closure will have to be structured with every session, as will the opportunity for discussion.

3. Assessment of Environmental Supports and Constraints

A. Facilities and materials

A wide range of activities can be conducted in the occupational therapy room and kitchen areas. The unit is not, however, large enough to accommodate group activities that require a lot of movement, physical sports equipment, or space.

B. Scheduling

Because of the other treatments scheduled, the hospital meal schedule, and patient visiting hours, the group meeting time is on a fixed schedule.

C. Group norms and prior therapy group experience (if any)

Physically or verbally abusive behaviors are not allowed on the unit. Patients who are unable to respect this requirement or require a locked unit for their own safety or the safety of others are referred to other facilities. Patients who do not participate in their treatment program, as established by the individual patients and staff, are terminated from the inpatient service. Patients who require long-term treatment on an inpatient unit are referred to other facilities. Alcohol and other nonprescribed drugs are not permitted on the unit. Smoking is permitted only in the community room (when therapy is not in session). Some members have had no prior therapy experience; others have participated in groups on prior admissions or in other facilities.

D. Do any of the environmental constraints require modification of the group, or could you alter the situation (such as locating needed materials)?

Under the leaders' supervision, the group could use the hospital grounds and surrounding areas for activities that require a lot of space and movement, such as sports.

General Group Plan Protocol

A Typical Group Protocol in the Design Stage

A. Name of Group   Project Group

B. Time/length of meeting(s)   Monday–Friday, 11:15–12:00 P.M.

C. Place   General Hospital Acute Psychiatric Inpatient Unit: Occupational Therapy Room

D. Open   X   or Closed Group

Statement of rationale:

Maximum length of stay is 4 weeks; average length of stay is 8 to 10 days; 16-bed unit.

E. Group Goals:

Depending on the specific group, these may include primary and secondary objectives and leader objectives for group as a whole and/or individual members.

1. Goals (behaviors you wish to increase or decrease)

To be able to contribute ideas, in the group, for the selection of a group project.

To be able to carry out selected aspects of the group project in the presence of others in the group, for example, get and distribute materials to group members.

To be able to verbally express satisfaction about one's own interaction in the group, contribution to the project, and the group's final product.

To be able to assume group maintenance roles such as encourager, compromiser, and gatekeeper. For example, make statements such as: "Let's try it," "Can we do what some members want to do today and what the rest want to do tomorrow?" or "Let's not pick a theme until we hear every opinion in the group."

To be able to assume group task roles, such as asking for information, giving opinions, or expressing wishes.

2. Rationale for goal selection

On admission, members presented problems such as poor self-esteem; withdrawal from family, friends, or coworkers; loss of interest in avocational activities; indecisiveness regarding what was usually "routine" decision making; and an inability to complete tasks required for daily functioning, such as food shopping, physical care of children, and banking.

3. Outcome criteria for successful goal attainment in session(s) stated in behavioral terms

At least once in every session, each member gives or seeks information; follows through with an action step necessary for the completion of the group project; and laughs, jokes, or smiles.

F. Group Composition or Criteria for Selecting Members

Ideally, the group should include both men and women and a maximum of eight members. In addition, prospective candidates for the group should minimally be able to communicate verbally in a simple manner; understand simple communications, for example, written and verbal instructions; concentrate on a structured task within the presence of seven other patients and two therapists, for a minimum of 30 minutes; and understand the goals and methods of the Project Group.

It is expected that members will have a variety of occupational behavior problems. Usually, prospective group members have psychiatric conditions that influence their abilities to fulfill social needs; feel masterful or useful; and meet obligations of social roles such as parent, worker, community member, or player.

G. Leadership Roles and Functions

The Project Group has two leaders. Their primary roles and functions are to establish a group structure that encourages a high degree of membership involvement in the group's task and selected processes; to protect the safety of individual group members and the morale of the group as a whole; to encourage action within the range of member abilities and perceptions of such; to act as resource persons for the making of projects and elements of group process and dynamics; and to communicate knowledge of members' adaptive behaviors and maladaptive behaviors to the group and unit staff.

H. Characteristics of Group Contract

Members are expected to attend sessions on a regular basis unless unusual circumstances prevail and the leaders must be notified of such circumstances before the session in question. The members are also required to remain in each group session for 45 minutes or to negotiate with the group or leaders if a special contract or arrangement is necessary because of extenuating circumstances.

Material discussed by other group members is not to be shared outside of the psychiatric unit patients and staff. Neither physical nor verbal abuse is tolerated in the group. If members are unable to fulfill the requirements of the group contract, they will be terminated from the group.

I. Group Methods and Procedures to be Employed:

Description or listing of methods, techniques, and modalities
Graded structured activity

Group process and task analysis
Group process and task adaptation
Crafts, horticulture, expressive art, and cooking

CASE STUDY NUMBER 2
Closed Occupational Therapy Group

Group History

1. This group format has been offered at the occupational therapy clinic for the past year. The group consists of eight consecutive sessions over a 2-week period. The chief occupational therapist and chief physiatrist have ultimate authority over the group's goals and structure.

2. The group is voluntary and composed of a maximum of eight members. The members are patients at the Rehabilitation Hospital, are 17 years of age or older, include both men and women, and are to be discharged within 2 to 3 weeks. Patients referred to the group are those needing help with energy conservation, time management, and adjustment to a disability. The group is thus named the Energy Conservation/Time Management Group.

   The occupational therapist screens patients on physician or occupational therapist referral. Patients must be oriented, able to communicate verbally and understand oral instructions, relatively emotionally stable, and able to concentrate on a task for 60 minutes.

   The group was started because patients seen in the outpatient clinic expressed a need for more input and support during discharge. They found returning home very stressful, and complained of strained family and coworker relationships, fatigue, depression, anxiety, and feeling useless. In fact, the first of these groups was started as a peer support group, with the consultation of an occupational therapist. It later became institutionalized as part of the clinic program when the staff found that the patients in the support group required less follow-up care.

3. This is a closed group with required attendance. The group meets four times per week for 2 weeks.

4. The structure of the group includes eight units. These segments are sequenced to parallel and facilitate a group's phases of development. The group is intended to teach skills and at the same time develop into a group-centered, cohesive support group. The group leaders, the occupational therapists, have the power to change the group's structure as long as the goals remain the same in regards to discharge planning.

5. The group is developed along the model of a functional group.

Assessment of Members

1. **Assessment of Group Members (Including Range of Behaviors)**

   A. General description

   Seven adults ranging from 31 to 66 years of age. There are four women (two had cerebrovascular accidents, one has arthritis, and one has multiple sclerosis) and three men (one has alcoholism, one had a myocardial infarction, and one has chronic undifferentiated pain). All are mildly depressed or anxious. All members live in suburban areas and cities within a 2-hour drive of the hospital.

   B. General description of members' expected environment

   All members will return to live at home alone, with spouses, family members, or children. Two members are retired, two are homemakers, one is unemployed, one runs a small family business, and one is a teacher.

   C. Description of current performance in areas of occupational behavior

   Work: The range of member work skills includes full to partial homemaking skills, full employment potential to being unemployed with work potential (for example, functions at task independently for 60 minutes, held maintenance job for 3 years), and being retired and completely dependent on family with no interest in work.

   Self-care: The range of member self-care skills includes complete independence in physical daily living skills (namely, grooming and hygiene, feeding/eating, dressing, functional mobility, functional communication, and object manipulation) to partial dependence in small object manipulation, wheelchair mobility, transfers, functional ambulation, grooming/hygiene, and eating.

   Leisure: The range of member leisure skills includes recognition of avocational interests to no ability to identify activities or social situations that are perceived as playful or fun. All members express concern regarding their ability to adapt leisure activities, schedule, or home environment to enable participation in avocational pursuits. Many members have difficulty identifying community resources available for leisure activities.

   D. Cognitive behavior

   All members are able to concentrate on a task or concept for 60 minutes, are oriented to person, place, and time, and have immediate and recent memory. Range of insight varies from excellent to poor. Problem-solving ability ranges from being able to make decisions to total reliance on concrete cues for evaluating decisions and plans.

   E. Psychosocial behavior

   Most members seldom initiate conversation with individuals other than the staff or their own family members; all express concern and anxiety over their appearance and ability to be productive or loved.

   F. Physical and neuromotor behavior

Many members become restless and agitated when expected to perform an activity. Several members have various degrees of physical dysfunction from a stroke, arthritic condition, neuromuscular disorder, chronic pain, general lethargy, or disuse of body. The range of problems includes poor dexterity and incoordination in fine motor tasks or gait, limited active range of motion, fatigue or strain when using muscular force required for certain activities, poor sensory awareness and postural balance, and poor visual–spatial awareness.

G. What is the significance of these factors with regard to individual member goals and forming or planning the group or group session(s)?
To promote total participation, ideally the group should be composed of no more than eight members (men and women) and have two leaders (one man and one woman). The group will need to be advised on how to select relatively short-term activities with little complexity and opportunity for error. The leaders will need to assume an active role in adapting the activities so that a variety of group membership roles can be practiced. They will also need to observe the group's process, suggest alternative behaviors, and assume group membership and leadership roles when the members are unable to do so. A highly supportive, genuine, and consistent emotional climate must be established and reinforced by the leaders.

2. **Assessment of Group Context (the Facility)**

    A. General description of program in which group is included (administrative structure)
    The group is one of the treatment services offered through the occupational therapy department to inpatients of the hospital. The leadership responsibility rotates among the occupational therapy staff of 18 certified therapists. Supervision is provided by the director of occupational therapy. Consultation services are also available from the staff physicians.

    B. General description of physical environment
    Large occupational therapy clinic with adapted kitchen, prevocational area, activity area with tables and chairs, and reception desk and offices in foyer of clinic space. The clinic is wheelchair accessible.

    C. General description of emotional climate
    Cheerful, warm, friendly, relaxed, and supportive. Therapists are open and direct with patients.

    D. Frame of reference, purpose, and objectives
    Biopsychosocial/ecological; rehabilitation and prevention services in a private rehabilitation hospital.

    E. What is the significance of these factors in forming or planning the group or group session(s)?
    Because the clinic space is used by other therapists treating patients in one-to-one therapies, a room divider will be required, as will coordination of use of supplies and equipment with other staff therapists.

3. Assessment of Environment Supports and Constraints

A. Facilities and materials
All materials are within easy access. Audiovisual equipment will be borrowed from the hospital supply area.

B. Scheduling
The group is scheduled in the morning, during the busiest portion of patients' treatment schedules, so the leaders will need to make arrangements with head nurses who coordinate patient rehabilitation programs. Some patients will need transportation aides to bring them to and from the occupational therapy clinic.

C. Group norms and prior therapy group experience (if any)
None.

D. Do any of the environmental constraints require modification of the group or could you alter the situation (such as locating needed materials)?
The group time might be rescheduled to 4:00 to 5:00 PM when the occupational therapy clinic is least crowded and patients have more flexibility in their schedules.

General Group Plan Protocol

A Typical Group Protocol in the Design Stage

A. Name of Group   Energy Conservation/Time Management Group

B. Time/length of meeting(s)   9:00–10:00 AM eight consecutive sessions in 2 weeks

C. Place   Rehabilitation Hospital, Inpatient Services, Occupational Therapy Clinic

D. Open   or Closed Group   X

Statement of rationale:
This group is focused on issues related to discharge planning. It is therefore limited to patients who will be discharged in 2 to 3 weeks.

E. Group Goals:
Depending on the specific group, these may include primary and secondary objectives, leader objectives for group as a whole and/or individual members.

1. Goals (behaviors you wish to increase or decrease)

Leader objectives:
Evaluate performance problems related to occupational behaviors necessary for functioning in life roles.

Discharge planning:
Patient referral for outpatient/home treatment services.

Member objectives:

To identify changes in living environment and relationships necessary for adaptation to current disability. This includes the need for orthotics, prosthetics, and assistive/adaptive equipment, as well as the maintenance of such equipment and involvement of other individuals such as family members.

To identify potential barriers to adjustment to community living; for example, overindulgence of family members, architectural barriers, physical isolation, limited mobility, or emotional withdrawal of friends, family, lover, and coworkers.

To identify role changes necessary as a result of disability; for example, homemaker roles, work roles, or avocational roles.

To describe programs for intervening with potential barriers; for example, to be able to ask for help and receive help; to plan alternate routes and modifications of physical environment so that mobility is increased; to be able to give and receive feedback; to suggest compromises or alternatives.

To be able to prevent or minimize debilitation through organizing activities and schedule to minimize energy output.

To use joint protection and/or body mechanics principles to minimize stress on joints.

To be able to physically position self so that optimal functioning in life roles is feasible.

To be able to select, perform, and coordinate activity schedule to maintain a balance between rest, sleep, work, and leisure needs and interests.

To identify a peer support network in the community to aid adjustment to disability.

To describe abilities and strengths.

2. Rationale for goal selection

These goals were selected because the members' discharge environment involves dealing with changes in life roles such as asking other people to fulfill some needs (for example, personal care or care of usual responsibilities). It is also recognized that although members are expected to be functioning at maximum potential at discharge, they need strategies and support to physically, emotionally, and socially maintain themselves in the community. Similarly, patient education is necessary to prevent further debilitation or disability. Currently, patients have been observed to be highly dependent on staff to fulfill needs and interact on a parallel level with other patients in the hospital. Families of the patients have expressed concern over being able to cope with a disabled person at home.

3. Outcome criteria for successful goal attainment in session(s) stated in behavioral terms

Changes are made in member's home environment to accommodate or prevent further disability; for example, changes in furniture heights, and family member available to transport patient to work.

Members seek and offer assistance in group; share concerns in group; seek and offer suggestions in group.

Members conduct a meeting or phone friends, employer, or family while in hospital to discuss changes necessary to resuming or modifying role activities.

Members plan out a weekly schedule for postdischarge week, incorporating units of work, rest, play, and sleep equivalent to energy output level of predischarge week.

In doing group activities, members position themselves and protect their joints so that they can complete projects with minimal stress and at a maximal level of functioning.

Members have the telephone numbers of at least two individuals they can call for support when discharged from the hospital.

F. Group Composition or Criteria for Selecting Members
The group is composed of a maximum of eight men and women patients who are 17 years of age or older. Usual diagnoses include neurological disorders (such as stroke, multiple sclerosis, Guillain-Barré syndrome), arthritis, cardiac disease, alcoholism, and chronic pain. Patients must be ready for discharge within 2 to 3 weeks. They also should be oriented and able to concentrate on a task for 60 minutes, able to communicate verbally and understand oral instructions, and be relatively emotionally stable (in other words, not emotionally labile or a potential suicide risk).

G. Leadership Roles and Functions
Two leaders will conduct this group. The sessions are planned into eight units, designed and implemented by the group leaders. One leader will have responsibility for screening patient referrals and introductory interviews. The other leader will have responsibility for writing notes in the patients records and for making discharge plans. The responsibilities for these functions will rotate between the leaders after completion of an 8-unit group.

H. Characteristics of Group Contract
Members are required to attend all eight sessions. They must express an interest in sharing their concerns about discharge with other group members and be willing to participate in the group's activities. They must have prior permission and a referral from their attending physician.

I. Group Methods and Procedures to be Employed
Briefly describe or list methods, techniques, and modalities.

Session Number 1	Introduction to the group: a discussion of its purpose, goals, and procedures. Icebreaker exercise.
Session Number 2	Individual collages: group picks theme; group discussion.

Session Number 3	The "Pie of My Life" prehospitalization and posthospitalization: an expressive art activity. Discussion.
Session Number 4	Energy conservation: lecture, slide show, demonstration, practice, and discussion.
Session Number 5	Time management principles: lecture, problem-solving exercises, and discussion.
Session Number 6	Community resources: information and referrals. Dealing with human and architectural barriers: discussion, role play, and follow-up discussion.
Session Number 7	Activities configuration. Discussion.
Session Number 8	Establish resource network. Discuss termination, group review, and evaluation. Party.

Note. These plans would be modified according to the group's needs. For example, if the group has members of a predominant age, sex, functional impairment, or with common roles, the sessions would focus on issues related to these concerns.

CASE STUDY NUMBER 3
Community-Based Occupational Therapy Group

Group History

1. This is a new group that is to be formed for the first time. It is to be 10 weeks in duration. The members are to be senior citizens living in the community surrounding the senior center. The director of the center has contracted with the occupational therapist who will have direct responsibility for designing, implementing and evaluating the group.

2. The group leader has been hired to lead this group by the director of the senior center. The membership will be voluntary and composed of members currently attending the senior center who wish to join the group. The group has been described in general terms as designed for the frail elderly or those who may need support to engage in center activities.

3. The group will be a closed group of seven to nine members. It will meet 1 day a week for 1 1/2 hours.

4. Not applicable; a new group.

5. Not applicable; a new group.

Assessment of Members

1. Assessment of Group Members (Including Range of Behaviors)

   A. General description

   The group meets at the senior center, which is a community center for senior citizens in a suburban neighborhood. Center members are primarily local residents and come to the center from their homes. Education ranges from high school graduate to higher education. The members interviewed for this small group are frail elderly who have ongoing medical difficulties, which include various levels of dementia, and past history of stroke. One person has been receiving chemotherapy for cancer; and some are experiencing symptoms of grief and depression. Ages range from 70 to 90 years. The group is to have five women and two men.

   B. General description of members' expected environment

   Participants currently visit the senior center 1 or 2 days a week. Some live independently, others in the home of a relative. Roles include grandparent, parent, friend, community member, and family member.

   C. Description of current performance in areas of occupational behavior (according to observed behavior and information from interview)

   Work: Members are retired and do no paid work.

   Self-care: Members demonstrate a range of self-care ability from independent to partially dependent on assistance. Home health aides, relatives and/or household help assist with bathing, dressing and other personal needs. Meals are delivered to some members and others eat with their families. Transportation to the center is provided by friends, relatives, and occasionally by taxi or minibus.

   Leisure: Members arrive at the center between 9 and 10 AM. Some have tea or coffee which is provided for them by the center volunteers but few of them participate in center activities. They will be a part of the activity group. Information regarding use of leisure time and interests was vague. Most leisure activities are instigated by family members.

   D. Cognitive behavior

   Members appear to understand that the purpose of the interview is to seek membership in the new group. All are oriented to time, place, and person.

   E. Psychosocial behavior

   Two members appeared withdrawn at the time of the interview and most of the information was given by an accompanying relative. One member seemed confused and appeared to be having trouble with her hearing aid. Others appeared reluctant to initiate conversation although they appeared to understand the questions asked and their answers were appropriate.

F. Physical and neuromotor behavior

Members demonstrated various levels of ambulatory ability. Three used walkers, one a cane. Some have visual or hearing deficits. A few appeared to have fine motor coordination, strength and range of motion deficits. All members appeared to be able to maintain sufficient balance to perform tabletop activities.

G. What is the significance of these factors with regard to individual member goals and forming or planning the group or group session(s)?

Group leader will need to provide a group structure with activities as well as a safe climate while encouraging members to interact in the group. The leader will have to assume an active role in adapting activities and assume membership and leadership roles when members are unable to do so. A supportive, genuine, and consistent emotional climate will need to be established and reinforced by the leader.

2. Assessment of Group Context (the Facility)

A. General description of program in which group is included (administrative structure)

The senior center is a community-based center for senior citizens. It is funded from grant money, city funds, and private funds. There is a board of directors that oversees the administration of the center. There is an administrator who makes policy and administrative decisions in conjunction with the board. The administrator is a social worker who is directly responsible for staff selection and the program. It is the administrator, in consultation with the board, who engaged the occupational therapist to lead the new group and negotiated the funds for her salary. The center is assisted by a dedicated group of volunteers who lead groups and activities and help in the day-to-day functions of the center.

B. General description of physical environment

The senior center is a modern, two-story building with a large recreation room, kitchen and eating area, and meeting rooms on the first floor. Offices and additional meeting rooms are located on the second floor. There is a large parking lot in the back that provides direct ground level entrance to the center. In the room where the group will meet there are cupboards, a sink, and a solid table on which to work. The room is well lighted with a row of windows on one wall. The activity room is adjacent to the recreational room and easily accessible for walkers, wheel chairs, etc.

C. General description of emotional climate

The general climate at the center is friendly and warm. Members are supportive of one another in particular. The objective is to help participants remain independent and living in their home environment where they are the happiest and where the quality of their lives is maximized.

D. Frame of reference, purpose, and objectives

The purpose of the center is to meet the ongoing needs of community residents; senior citizens in particular.

E. What is the significance of these factors for forming or planning the group or group session(s)?

The structure of the senior center allows for the creation of a weekly closed group where the same participants come every Wednesday morning. A review of the group structure and process will be done weekly.

3. Assessment of Environmental Supports and Constraints

A. Facilities and materials

It is possible to carry out a wide range of activities while sitting around the table in the meeting room. Other rooms might be available should more space be required. Materials are available for the group in the cupboard and special purchases can be made as needed. An assistant to the group leader will be available from the group of experienced volunteers and time will be allowed for the volunteer aide and the leader to plan and discuss the group sessions. The volunteer aide has agreed to attend the group consistently for 10 weeks.

B. Scheduling

This group is scheduled to meet on Wednesday mornings from 10:00 to 11:30 AM in the activity room. The length of time has been selected to give participants ample time to complete the short-term activities without feeling hurried and pressed for time.

C. Group norms and prior therapy group experience (if any)

All participants will attend this group voluntarily. They will be encouraged to attend and participate fully. Physical or verbally abusive behaviors will not be acceptable. Smoking is not permitted in the center.

D. Do any of the environmental constraints require modification of the group, or could you alter the situation (such as locating needed materials)?

None at present.

General Group Plan Protocol

A Typical Group Protocol in the Design Stage

A. Name of Group: Activity Group

B. Time/length of meeting(s): Wednesday, 10:00–11:30 AM

C. Place: Senior Center Activity Room

D. Open   X   or Closed Group

Statement of rationale:

To limit the number of participants and to have a stable group of similar abilities.

E. Group Goals:

Depending on the specific group, these may include primary and secondary objectives and leader objectives for group as a whole and/or individual members.

1. Goals (behaviors you wish to increase or decrease)

To verbally interact with other group members.

To actively participate in group activities.

To contribute ideas to the selection of group activities.

To relax and enjoy oneself in group activities.

2. Rationale for goal selection

Members are either at risk of or experience social isolation.

Members manifest various levels of decreased life-role performance; decreased ability and competence in the areas of physical, cognitive and psychosocial performance.

3. Outcome criteria for successful goal attainment in session(s) stated in behavioral terms

During each session, each member will contribute verbally to the group at least once by expressing his or her thoughts to another group member or commenting about the group activity.

Members will take steps to help complete the group activity.

Members will show their pleasure/comfort level in the group by smiling or showing signs of decreased tension.

F. Group Composition or Criteria for Selecting Members

Group consists of five females and two males. Prospective members must express voluntary desire to join the group. Participants are chosen by the group leader based on their interest and their level of physical and psychosocial abilities.

G. Leadership Roles and Functions

The group is composed of a leader and one volunteer assistant who will plan and evaluate the group activities together. The volunteer assistant has made a commitment to consistently attend the group for the 10 weeks. The leader seeks to encourage suggestions and input from members in planning activities and sessions. Leaders seek member involvement by encouraging and modeling desired group behavior, i.e., listening, verbally participating, being supportive, and giving feedback. While maintaining the group structure, the leader will seek to adapt to the changing needs and dynamics of the group. Leaders will allow the group the freedom to grow and evolve within a safe and caring environment.

H. Characteristics of Group Contract

Participants, once they have been chosen, are expected to attend and participate in the group activities each week for 10 weeks. Leaders and members are expected to keep conversations confidential when away from the group.

I. Group Methods and Procedures to be Employed:

Briefly describe or list methods, techniques and modalities.

Structured group tasks within range of member ability.
Group process and task modification.
Simple structured interactive activities.
Crafts, role validation activities, and life review/reminiscence activities.
Group guidance for the discussion of action in the present.

Review Questions

1. What is meant by a group plan? Why is it needed in the design stage?
2. To promote adaptation through occupation the group progresses through four successive interdependent stages. What are these stages?
3. Why is the leader role in the design stage important to the group's ultimate success?
4. What are the five leader functions of the design stage?
5. What is meant by a "group contract"? Who are the individuals involved in creating a group contract?
6. What is meant by a "flow experience" and how may this be achieved?

References

Barris, R., Kielhofner, G., and Watts, J. H. (1983). Psychosocial Occupational Therapy: Practice in a Pluralistic Arena. Laurel, MD: Ramsco.

Csikszentmihalyi, M. (1975). Beyond Boredom and Anxiety: The Experience of Play in Work and Games. San Francisco: Jossey-Bass.

Hemphill, B. J. (ed.) (1982). The Evaluative Process in Psychiatric Occupational Therapy. Thorofare, NJ: Charles B. Slack.

Mosey, A. C. (1973). Activities Therapy. New York: Raven Press.

Persson, D. (1996). Play and flow in an activity group—a case study of creative occupations with chronic pain patients. Scandinavian Journal of Occupational Therapy 3:33–42.

Yalom, I. D. (1970). The Theory and Practice of Group Psychotherapy. New York: Basic Books.

Yalom, I. D. (1983). Inpatient Group Psychotherapy. New York: Basic Books.

Chapter 7
Stage Two: Formation

Events which strengthen bonds between members enhance the potency of the group. (YALOM, 1975, p. 120)

- **Group Actions**
- Purposeful Action
- Self-Initiated Action
- Spontaneous Action
- Group-Centered Action

  Leader Functions and Intervention Strategies
  Setting the Climate
  Clarifying Goals and Norms
  Selecting Purposeful Action
  Leader Emotional Response

  Conclusion
  CASE STUDY NUMBER 1: Open Occupational Therapy Group
  "Breaking the Ice": A Typical Group Session in the Formation Stage
  CASE STUDY NUMBER 2: Closed Occupational Therapy Group
  A Problematic Group Session in the Formation Stage
  CASE STUDY NUMBER 3: Community-Based Occupational Therapy Group
  A Senior Activity Group in the Formation Stage

  Review Questions

  References

The formation stage of a group begins at the first meeting. This event is marked by a combination of anticipation and apprehension on the part of the leader and the members. The predominant processes during the initial sessions of the group involve orientation and exploration by all participants as members get acquainted, learn how the group functions, and develop norms that will shape their behavior in the group. They may also explore their own hopes and fears about the group situation and try to formulate their personal goals. They may deal with issues of feeling "in" or "out" of the group, perhaps even make a decision to stay in the group and get involved or to leave. The manner in which the leader deals with these behaviors will, to a large extent, determine the degree of trust and cohesiveness that will be present at any time during the life of the group.

The specific aspects of the group that characterize the formation stage include:

- personal feelings of belonging and acceptance
- dependence on the leader and testing the leadership
- individual versus group goals
- trust versus mistrust

These are listed here roughly in the order in which they arise in many groups, but the order may vary according to the design of the particular group. Each of these aspects will be discussed in this chapter in relation to the characteristics of the actions of the functional group (Table 7-1). These actions are as follows:

- the purposeful (task) action
- the self-initiated action
- the spontaneous or "here-and-now" action
- the group-centered action

The features of the initial sessions of a group may also be pertinent to the starting phases of individual group meetings. Each separate meeting is a microcosm of a series of group sessions; each meeting passes through the stages of formation, development, and termination. The starting segments of individual group sessions commonly exhibit the characteristics of the early group meetings. It is not unusual for a group to spend the final minutes of a meeting planning for the next meeting and then to spend the initial period of the subsequent meeting altering the previously made plans. Establishing control over the group's functioning is one of the group-centered actions that develop during the formation stage of the group.

Group Actions

Each of the four types of action of the functional group serves to facilitate the achievement of the members' ultimate goals. Also, each involves a response to the four issues related to this stage.

Purposeful Action

The purposeful action of the formation stage in the functional group can contribute directly to the feelings of acceptance and belonging of group development. All members need to be included and to participate in the group action. Eric Berne (1963) wrote, "The principle concern of every healthy group is to survive as long as possible, or at least until the task is done" (p. 77). For a group to work together on a task, individuals must be drawn together as members in the group, and individuals will be drawn to a group that promises to meet their needs and interests (Box 7-1). Because the prospect of success also increases group attractiveness, the activity must be carefully matched with the skill level of the participants so members can expect a successful outcome. The leader must seek opportunities to guide the action at the proper level of challenge for the group members, thereby creating a "flow experience."

Table 7-1
Group Membership Needs Related to Action: Formation Stage

Formation Stage Issues	Purposeful Action	Self-Initiated Action
Concern over belonging and acceptance	Action that includes all members 1) Structured 2) Successful outcome for all	Acceptance of "polite" social behavior Support for expression of negative and positive feelings
Dependence on leader	Strong leader involvement in task selection and adaptation	Leader encouragement of exploratory role
Testing leader style	Guidance regarding expectations of member roles	Behavior risk taking
Clarification of individual and group goals	Clear options and alternatives in goal selection An accepting climate	Expression of individual goals Behavior risk taking
Testing for trust	Respect for opinions and feelings of members An accepting climate	Group support and encouragement for individual roles and goals Behavior risk taking

Spontaneous (Here-and-Now) Action	Group-Centered Action	Leader Skills Employed
Encouragement of expression of ideas, feelings, and thoughts related to here-and-now action	Established pattern Beginning knowledge of group resources Gradual sharing by members in leadership	Analysis and adaptation of interaction Genuineness and empathy, listening and responding
Opportunity to interact with leader and to test degree of freedom and control	Leader input as needed Leader support Examination of group goals and exploration	Modeling Tentativeness Feedback Sharing rationale for leader action
Sharing of member perceptions and reactions as to what is going on in the group	of norms appropriate to reaching group goals Group-centered decision-making process	Genuineness and empathy, listening and responding Concreteness Classification
Experience support and acceptance of diversity	Developing concensus	Genuineness and empathy, listening, and responding Climate setting for supportive interpersonal relationships
Sharing of member perceptions and re-actions to what is going on in the group	Awareness of group's own process	Discussing confidentiality Structuring action for member comfort and growth Genuineness and empathy, listening and responding

> Box 7-1
> **Strong Beginning**
>
> The purposeful action of the beginning group must be an activity that will interest and ensure the participation of the members.

Member acceptance and belongingness are also increased when the purposeful action of the formative stage provides a fair amount of structure. A clear structure helps new members recognize quickly and easily what behavior is desirable in the group; this, in turn, helps them to feel more comfortable. A structured task supplies the members with clearly defined roles, goals, and limits, thus reducing member anxiety. For example, a common activity in a new group is an exercise called an icebreaker. The action goal of this exercise is to help members learn everyone's names and to establish contact and communication with each other. The directions are simple and clear. All members participate according to the structure of the particular exercise, and member interaction is achieved.

The specific purposeful action of the group influences the degree of authority the leader holds in the group. When the activity is structured, the leader holds an authoritative role; when the task is less structured, the members hold more authority than the leader, leaving them to exercise more control over their actions. The purposeful action (or task) thereby regulates the degree of dependence or independence exhibited by members in the group. By the choice of a task, the leader can influence the extent to which members will function independently or dependently.

Similarly, the purposeful action of the formative stage aids the inclusion of both group and individual goals. The character of the purposeful action provides the structure for reaching specific goals, and through participation in selected tasks, the group establishes and clarifies its goals.

The manner of carrying out purposeful action is also closely associated with the level of trust or mistrust in the formative stage of the functional group. When the comfort level of the group is high, trust is enhanced. When the comfort level of the group is low, mistrust is common. Further, a task successfully completed enhances trust. Members usually start to give each other feedback, both positive and negative, on aspects of the purposeful action of the group. As the group begins to acknowledge this type of feedback and act on it, group trust and cohesiveness develop. The leader can teach members how to give and receive feedback constructively through the example that he or she provides.

Self-Initiated Action

After an initial introduction by the leader and a brief synopsis of the general goals of the group, a period of dramatic silence usually ensues as members become anxious and do not know how to respond. The early sessions are characterized by the members' uncertainty over how to behave (Box 7-2). For example, members will seek acceptance through polite social conversation. Members who feel awkward during moments of silence will seek to keep the conversation flowing on almost any topic. Other members who feel most comfortable with action will become impatient to get started on any kind of group task or activity and will make comments about their activity interests.

Member self-initiated action in the formation stage is usually directed toward the leader. Members in the functional group—commonly patients in treatment programs—feel highly dependent on the leader for guidance toward personal therapeutic goals at the outset. They see the leader as a figure of authority and the patient as a person who complies with that authority. Frequently, members look to the leader to make them feel comfortable and to reduce their anxiety and discomfort. When these hopes are not realized, resistance and hostility may be directed toward the leader. It is common for members of new groups to direct their statements to the group leader rather than to their fellow members. As time goes on, leader dependence may shift to the opposite extreme of counterdependence. Members may display resistance to leadership, becoming highly suspicious of the leader and afraid of being manipulated. This resistance may be manifested in dissatisfaction with details about the arrangements for the group, such as the time or place of group meetings.

Once members are acquainted, self-initiated action takes a different form. Gradually, questions about group goals emerge, and members begin to discuss, clarify, and develop goals. Through taking risks and verbalizing personal fears or perceptions about what is happening in the group, members help build a climate of trust. According to Carl Rogers (1969), "If this self-initiated learning is to occur, it seems essential that the individual be in contact with, be faced by, a real problem. Success in facilitating such learning often seems directly related to this factor" (pp. 58–59).

Spontaneous Action

At first, there is little spontaneity as members seek acceptance through polite conversation about current or past events. Members' listening skills are usually poor, and an exchange of ideas may be difficult. Suggestions are made, but there are few respondents to support or explore them. As time passes, positive and

Box 7-2
Early Stages

The period of self-initiated action commonly takes the form of polite, stereotypic social behavior.

negative opinions are verbalized, and as these opinions are supported a climate of respect for the feelings and opinions of individual group members develops. From his extensive experience with groups, Carl Rogers (1970) states, "Curiously enough, the first expression of genuinely here and now feeling is apt to come out in negative attitudes towards other group members or towards the leader. Frequently the leader is attacked for failure to give proper guidance to the group" (p. 18).

The issue of dependence on and independence from the leader is highlighted throughout the here-and-now action stage (Box 7-3). On the basis of their group experience, members realize that the leader neither answers all their needs nor makes all decisions. As the leader refers tasks to the group, members learn to be less reliant on the leader. They begin to test the amount of freedom and control they can manage within the setting of the group (Fig. 7-1). They also begin to feel more comfortable with group silences and learn to tolerate them with less anxiety.

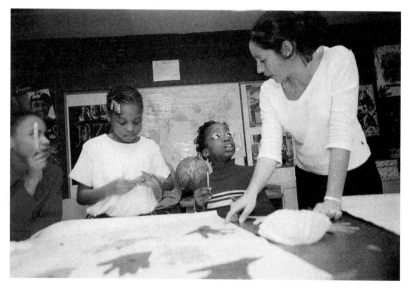

Figure 7-1. Establishing group-centered action: Independence and dependence on the leader. (Photograph by Sarah Brezinsky.)

The process of establishing norms and goals in a group helps the group interact in the here-and-now context because norms refer to immediate concerns. Immediacy gives impetus to a genuine exploration of conflicts and problems as members share their own reactions to what is happening in the group. Through interaction and sharing, members deal with individual concerns about being pressured or forced by the group to conform against their will or inclination. Within this spontaneous action, group trust can grow as individual members experience support and tolerance for diversity. The development of trust in the early stages of a group, according to Corey and Corey (1982), requires a climate of respect for the opinions and feelings of group members.

Group-Centered Action

As the formative stage of the group progresses, group-centered action develops. As members begin to feel a sense of belonging and acceptance, a climate of respect for the individual emerges, and members become better listeners and communicators. This climate encourages members to assume more leadership roles; in some instances, members may even challenge the leader. As the leader relinquishes some of his or her responsibility to the group members, the members and the leader develop a different relationship. Interdependence develops as the group works out new procedures, norms, and values appropriate to reaching its goals and using its resources. Interdependence in this context is defined as learning to accept dependence when it is truly needed and relying on leader and member expertise to help the group to function.

In their research on early group decisions, Gibb and Gibb (1967) observed that at the beginning of the formation stage, poor decision making is characteristic of group-centered action. As the emotional and social needs of the members are met and the group develops norms of individual support, members begin to restate and reexamine the group goals, taking the necessary time to seek every member's opinion and establish a group consensus. These group-centered activities contribute to an atmosphere of trust, and it is not uncommon at this point to find members raising issues of confidentiality to test the degree of group trust.

The ultimate goal of the formation stage is to achieve a "psychological

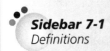

Sidebar 7-1
Definitions

Interdependence: *Learning to accept dependence when it is truly needed, and relying on leader and member expertise to help the group function*

Psychological group: *The ultimate goal of the formation stage*

Group climate: *The ongoing attitudes and concepts that pervade the group*

group." According to Bradford (1978), a psychological group forms under specific conditions:

- Patterns of interaction are proven effective
- Differences in perceptions about task, communication, and procedures are clarified
- Relationships to other persons and groups are delineated
- Standards for participation are set
- Methods of work that elicit rather than inhibit member contributions are established
- A respected "place" for each person is secured
- Trust is established among members (p. 5)

Leader Functions and Intervention Strategies

The four group actions described earlier are initiated and directed by the leader. In this section, we consider the role of the group leader in the formation stage and present strategies for effective leader participation. Two primary issues of the formation stage are members' need for acceptance and the development of relationships with the group leader. The group leader can facilitate these processes through specific strategies.

Setting the Climate

As the organizer of the group, the leader sets the climate. The term *group climate* refers to the ongoing attitudes and concepts that pervade the group. Apart from specific strategies, the leader's interpersonal style will, to some extent, influence the group climate. The warmth and acceptance of the leader and the ability to convey respect for each member contribute to a supportive group climate. In their report of research studies of therapy groups, Truax and Mitchell (1971) wrote that a supportive and empathetic relationship with the leader is positively correlated with member progress in treatment. They also report that there is a significant positive correlation between the degree of support offered by the leader and group member outcome; that is, the more support offered by the leader, the better the results achieved by the members.

During the early group sessions, while members search for acceptable behavior in the group, they are dependent on the leader for guidance. Both openly through their statements and covertly through their actions, they look to the leader for direction and structure, as well as approval. The leader may well wonder how much structure should be provided at this point. Yalom (1983) favors a middle ground between too much structure and too little structure:

> Although patients desire and require considerable structuring by the therapist, excessive structure may retard their therapeutic growth. If the leader does everything for patients, they will do little for themselves. Thus, in the early stages of therapy, structure provides reassurance to the frightened and confused patient; but persistent and rigid structure, over the long run, can infantalize the patient and delay assumption of autonomy. (p. 123)

Box 7-4
Leader Options

The leader of the functional group can reduce the importance of the leader role by assuming the role of a consultant or troubleshooter.

It seems that although members like the leader who provides the greatest structure, they are less likely to achieve therapeutic changes when working with such a leader.

One of the roles of the leader is to teach members to assume responsibility for themselves and their group. This can be accomplished by sharing the rationale for leader actions with the members. By modeling certain behaviors, the leader can also teach members to increase their participation through a variety of roles. This method of teaching was presented in some detail in Chapter 5 (Box 7-4). The leader can support the members in a variety of ways. According to Yalom (1983):

> The therapist supports by treating the patient with respect and dignity. The therapist supports by identifying and reinforcing the patient's strengths and virtues. The therapist supports by refraining from undermining defenses but instead by bolstering them and by encouraging patients to employ defenses that are at least one step more effective than the one they are currently using. (p. 128)

The leader should create a climate that is experienced as constructive and supportive, one in which members feel safe and can learn to trust the group. Genuine trust takes time and hard work. Members cannot trust each other unless they know each other, respect one another, and believe that they will be listened to and that a sincere attempt will be made to understand them. Trust grows from working and learning together. A group may be successful but still not achieve trust among its members.

Clarifying Goals and Norms

The group leader should state the purposes and goals of the group at the first session. Leaders may also wish to express personal feelings, hopes, and expectations that they have for the group. For instance, the leader of a group may begin with the following statement. "In this group we are going to work hard and at the same time have some fun together. We will meet every Wednesday from 10:00 AM to noon in this room, and I expect you to attend all meetings. From time to time, new members will join the group. We are going to learn to plan group meetings together and then to complete the tasks that we have planned. This group is meeting to help you with your social relationships so that you can learn to interact more appropriately in your work situation or with your family. I am looking forward to being part of this group, to getting to know you, and to working with you to achieve our goals." The leader may then pause and invite member reactions and comments. Although the goals as stated may be clear to the leader, they may not be clear to the members. Members should be encouraged to ask questions and make comments.

Through this introductory statement, the leader has established specific norms for group behavior. First, the group can talk about its goals, task, and the perceptions of its members. Second, the leader will participate in this process. Third, the responsibility for planning and learning will be a total group responsibility. Fourth, regular group attendance will be expected, and this is an open group where new members may be expected. Finally, it is all right for members to have fun in the group.

If the leader continues to model the established norms as the group progresses, it will help the group create a safe climate for learning that will form the basis for group effectiveness. Napier and Gershenfeld (1983) present a list of norms that the leader can encourage. They are adapted here for the leader of the functional group:

1. *People should be listened to and recognized.* The leader should acknowledge a questioning look or tentative statement. The norm of personal respect and equal rights of membership in the group is established.
2. *The group is a safe place.* Members are reassured that what happens in the group stays within the group. A member will not be ridiculed or reprimanded for speaking out. The leader's behavior can be discussed just like any other point of discussion in the group. The leader will encourage quiet members to speak more often and talkative members to speak less often.
3. *Feelings are important.* The leader encourages the expression of feelings and establishes the norm that the expression of feelings is vital if the group is to use its energy toward resolving problems and reaching its goals.
4. *Objectivity is encouraged.* The group learns that when the leader asks for information from members or asks if others have similar feelings to those expressed, those feelings are not dismissed or smoothed over as nonexistent. The leader encourages observers and observation to demonstrate that all members can look at what is happening in the group.
5. *Members learn from doing things and analyzing them.* In the process of achieving the goals of the group, focusing on "here and now" is a major learning method.
6. *Planning is a joint effort.* The leader is involved with the members in planning for group sessions. The leader does not have sole responsibility for the success of the group.

These norms, established through the leader's actions, provide examples that influence the behavior of the members and invite members to participate in various group roles.

Clarifying goals, both group goals and individual goals, is crucial in the early stages of the group (Box 7-5). As the group gains experience, members become better able to formulate goals. Through their involvement helping others to identify ways of learning from the group, members get a better idea of how they, too, can profit from the group experience, and they thus become more adept at stating personal goals. At this point, the leader may be able to help members to develop contracts with the group as a method of reaching their personal goals. A contract is a statement made by the member to the group regarding what he or

> **Box 7-5**
> **Goal Clarification**
>
> Clarifying goals is an ongoing process throughout the life of the group, not something that is done only once at the outset.

she is willing to do during a group session or even outside of the group meeting. This contract states specific behaviors the member is willing to explore or change. Through the contract, the member assumes responsibility for his or her behavior and takes an active role in personal behavioral change.

Selecting Purposeful Action

A primary purpose of the formation stage is to assist members to feel accepted and included as valued members of the group; therefore, a purposeful action needs to be carefully selected and adapted by the leader. In discussing the planning stage of the group (see Chapter 6), the leader was advised to evaluate the level of member skills. It is particularly important in the early session of the group that the leader selects group tasks in which all members are assured of experiencing success. Again, the tasks should also be appealing to all group members. Finally, the purposeful action of the group sessions should be selected for its ability to draw in all members, on both the real and the symbolic level.

The leader must decide how much control to exercise over the group. To what degree will the leader or the members be in control? The relative importance of control will vary according to the characteristics of the members. Control is a major problem for some individuals, and tasks must be chosen by the leader with this problem in mind. External forms of regulation can be provided or diminished, often calibrated by choice versus nonchoice, structure versus lack of structure, imposed rules versus freedom, and so forth. For instance, if a group of adolescents has trouble accepting adult leadership, the leader should select a task with limits and controls that are inherent in that particular task. Through varied task selection and adaptation, the group leader can adjust the amount of control needed by the group to enable it to reach treatment goals.

Leader Emotional Response

Leader concerns in the group's formation may, just as in other stages, mirror member's emotional preoccupations. Fear of not being accepted or not belonging to the group is often a feeling experienced by members joining a newly forming group or an existing group. Questions about the purpose of the group and concerns about safety are common. These reactions may be unconscious

---

Box 7-6
Leader Self-Reflective Questions

- How do I react when excluded from a group?
- In what circumstances do I find that my behavior is overbearing or that I have difficulty asserting myself and attempt to please?
- Do I find myself attracted to people who overly depend on me? When might this become problematic as a group leader?
- Do I find myself more comfortable with individuals who resist authority? When might this become problematic as a group leader?
- What resources are available to me in learning more about myself or developing skills such as being more assertive, for example, counseling groups or peer supervision groups?

---

or misunderstood by the members. They can take the form of testing the leader and dependence on the leader.

As strong reactions emerge in a group, as explained earlier, it is not uncommon for the leader to also experience concerns similar to group members. They too may fear lack of acceptance by the group and loss of members. If these feelings are unexamined or unacknowledged, the therapist is in danger of acting out. For example, the therapist may unwittingly be too loose and not establish enough structure around group norms such as being on time. Likewise, they might overly regulate boundaries and be extremely rigid. Self-reflective questions can help leaders to self-examine their emotional responses and to identify patterns in their own reactions to working in the formation stage (Box 7-6). The Group Session Plan Protocol and Session Evaluation Form (see Case Studies 1, 2, and 3 in the Formation Stage) can help the leader reason about and select an appropriate structure to address these concerns.

Conclusion

Analysis of the types of behavior that may appear in this stage should indicate that the leader has a variety of techniques and strategies available to guide the group members as they begin their work as a group but also that the leader cannot completely control the group behavior. Leaders must expect and prepare for certain standard behavior patterns adopted by individuals confronted with an entirely new set of circumstances. Careful planning in the use of resources and leadership skills will enable the leader to build a cohesive and functioning group.

In the following pages, we continue with our case studies by including complete protocols for sessions and evaluations for the open and closed groups in the formation stage. These case studies provide the reader with concrete examples of functional group work.

Open Occupational Therapy Group

"Breaking the Ice": A Typical Group Session in the Formation Stage

Group Session Plan Protocol

A. Name of Group   Project Group

Date   June 6

B. Specific goals for the group session
Given a leader-structured and directed task, members are:
To learn other group members' names.
To talk to another group member and the group as a whole.
To take turns talking in a group.

C. Specific goals for group members if different from those just listed and goals for each group member
Gary, Eric, Liz, and Pearl: To express their feelings and reactions to being members of a group with four incoming new members.
New group members: To decrease feelings of anxiety about being in the group and increase feelings of acceptance and belonging.

D. Description of and rationale for methods and procedures
Explain group goals, leader and member roles, group structure, and limits (to help members understand the purpose of the group's activities and to instill feelings of safety and belonging).
Describe icebreaker activity in simple and clear fashion (to decrease tension in group and help members feel less isolated).

E. Description of and rationale for leadership role
The leaders should optimally provide enough task structure and support so that members feel reassured that they are safe yet not be too rigid or directive as to encourage overly dependent behavior on the part of group members.

F. Describe necessary preparations
Review session plan among coleaders.
Gather supplies necessary for group activity.
Prepare new members for group in individual pregroup interviews.

G. List material and equipment needed
Eight pieces of 8 1/2 × 11 inch lined writing paper
Eight sharpened pencils with erasers
Pencil sharpener

H. Time and sequence outline for sessions, including what you will do and say as leader and what the group will do; consider both content and process.

Explain group's purpose, leader and member roles, and expectations (approximately 5 minutes).

Explain that because so many new members are in the group today, the leaders have planned an activity to help group members get to know one another. Pass out a piece of paper and pencil to each group member. Ask that everyone write down their first and last name on the top of the paper. Then explain that each person will first write down two things they like about their name and two things they might not like about their name. Explain that after completing this part of the activity, each member will share what they have written down on the paper with the person sitting to the right of him or her. Once everyone has completed this part of the activity, members will take turns introducing their partner by sharing what that person said they did and did not like about their name. The group is told that members will be encouraged to talk about their reactions to this activity afterward (approximately 5 minutes).

The group will then do the described activities. The leaders will encourage member participation, keep group activity within time limits of session by prompting group to complete various aspects of task, and clarify directions as needed (approximately 25 minutes).

Leaders will summarize the group's purpose and discuss potential plans for the following session with group members (approximately 10 minutes).

I. **Other information pertinent to this specific session:**
For example: Will there be any new members, coleaders, or guests? Is there an unusual tone on the unit or special event that is about to occur or just occurred for the individual member or group?

In this session, half of the group will be composed of new members.

Session Evaluation Form Protocol

A. **Name of Group**   Project Group

Date   June 6

B. **Were the goals accomplished? (Give rationale and state outcome.)**
Partially. Gary had difficulty taking turns speaking in group and interrupted several times while other group members were talking. Bette, a new group member, remained in the group for 10 minutes and left saying she was too "nervous" to sit any longer. All other members accomplished the session goals.

Was the session helpful in accomplishing short-term and long-term group and individual member goals?
Yes, except for Bette (see previous statement).

Do you have any evidence that the session(s) have been helpful to the members' functioning (adaptation) outside of the group?
Yes. The leaders have observed group members informally chatting on the unit at lunch.

C. Was the group structure adequate for accomplishing the goals? Give rationale and consider: leadership; time/length of meeting; open vs. closed group; time, sequence, methods and procedures; media/modalities/techniques employed; norms/behaviors reinforced implicitly or explicitly; methods of reinforcement; and stage of group's development.

Partially. For most of the group members, the structure established a nonthreatening climate.

Did the structure prove optimal "action" or "flow activity" for a "flow state" to occur?

Yes. For the most part, members interacted in a spontaneous manner when paired with another member. However, the leaders should take on more directive roles during future group discussions.

Did the structure provide optimal purposeful, self-initiated, spontaneous, and group-centered "action" for cognitive and emotional impact, skill learning, and adaptation to occur through "occupation"?

Given the group's stage of development, the structure did encourage members to interact in an optimal fashion. Hence, with leader input, the members completed the structured group task.

Did the structure provide for new learning, reinforcement of current level of functioning, or adaptation, or did it reinforce functioning below current level of adaptation? Explain and give rationale.

The structure encouraged all members to learn the value of sharing concerns in a group. Except for Bette, the range of group processes enabled members to participate at a parallel through cooperative level.

Did the structure provide an opportunity for evaluation and feedback regarding the group procedures and member progress? Explain.

Yes. Members were encouraged to discuss their reactions to the session and ideas for future sessions. The leaders had ample opportunity to observe member behavior/reactions to varying degrees of task structure.

D. What changes would you make in group goals and structure for the next session, or if you were to lead this session again?

In the event that an uneven number of members is remaining in a group, I would avoid group activities requiring dyads.

E. Were you adequately prepared for the session? (Give rationale, considering such things as time, place, materials, and physical and emotional environment.)

Yes. Knowing there would be four new members was essential to the preparations, including planning a structured exercise.

F. How did you function as leader? How did your behavior and role affect the group? Were you effective? (Give rationale.) What did you learn about yourself as group leader?

When Gary had difficulty taking turns and Bette said she was leaving the group, I had to assume the group maintenance roles. Members responded by imitation and began to encourage each other to listen and share. I believe this was effective because it helped to model group norms and encouraged group-centered participation.

G. Was the group interaction as you anticipated? If problems occurred, what processes can you identify as a basis for understanding the problems?
I did not anticipate that Bette would have difficulty remaining in the group. The expectation that she remain in the group for 45 minutes appeared to overwhelm her.

H. In the future, what might you do differently as group leader? (Give rationale.)
I would speak with the nursing staff before the session to establish if any special events occurred before the session. Based on this information, I might make alternate agreements ("contracts") with patients who "need" to grade the amount of time spent in the group. For example, Bette could have been told she could stay in the group for 15 minutes the first time, 30 minutes the second, and so on, thereby encouraging success and establishing helpful limits.

CASE STUDY NUMBER 2
Closed Occupational Therapy Group

A Problematic Group Session in the Formation Stage

Group Session Plan Protocol

A. Name of Group   Energy Conservation/Time Management Group

Date   December 15, second session out of eight

B. Specific goals for the group session
To learn value of peer support and group problem solving.

C. Specific goals for group members if different from those just listed, and goals for each group member
Leader goal: to encourage group cohesiveness.

D. Description of and rationale for methods and procedures
Group discussion
Expressive art activity
Rationale: to increase trust, member sharing, and goal setting by establishing an environment that fosters free expression of common concerns.

E. Description of and rationale for leadership role
Encourage expression of fears and perceptions in here and now.
Clarify group goals and task.

Rationale: to enable group to establish a balance of group and individual goals and ensure that the group is a safe place to express concerns.

F. Describe necessary preparations
Gather art materials.

G. List material and equipment needed
Magazines, glue, scissors, large construction paper, tape, and a variety of precut magazine pictures

H. Time and sequence outline for session, including what you will do and say as leader and what the group will do; consider both content and process
   1. Introduce group to activity: state purpose, goals, and methods (approximately 5 minutes).
   2. Encourage group members to pick a group theme for the individual collages they will make. Explain the theme might be about, for example, discharge from the hospital. Assume group maintenance and task roles as needed by group (approximately 10 minutes).
   3. Members make collages with leader assistance/adaptation as necessary. Members are encouraged to help each other and ask for help when needed (approximately 30 minutes).
   4. Encourage members to share perceptions regarding the group theme and its relationship to their collages and the group's goals (approximately 15 minutes).

I. Other information pertinent to this specific session: for example: Will there be any new members, coleaders, or guests? Is there an unusual tone on the unit or special event that is about to occur or just occurred for the individual member or group?
None.

Session Evaluation Form Protocol

A. Name of Group   Energy Conservation/Time Management Group

   Date   December 15

B. Were the goals accomplished? (Give rationale and state outcome).
Partially. Members expressed their individual fears about discharge; however, only one or two members saw the value of the group for support or relevance of group goals.

Was the session helpful in accomplishing short-term and long-term group and individual member goals?
Yes. For members to establish trust and a feeling of belonging to the group, it is necessary that a balance between individual member and group goals be negotiated and tested in the group.

Do you have any evidence that the session(s) have been helpful to the members' functioning (adaptation) outside of the group?
No.

C. Was the group structure adequate for accomplishing the goals? Give rationale and consider leadership; time/length of meeting; open vs. closed group; time, sequence, methods and procedures; media/modalities/techniques employed; norms/behaviors reinforced implicitly or explicitly; methods of reinforcement; and stage of group's development.

The value of the group activity was not easily apparent to members. A more structured goal setting activity is preferable for this stage of the group's development.

Did the structure provide optimal "action" or "flow activity" for a "flow state" to occur?

No. Members needed more time to talk about their individual concerns.

Did the structure provide optimal purposeful, self-initiated, spontaneous, and group-centered "action" for cognitive and emotional impact, skill learning, and adaptation to occur through "occupation"?

No. As typical of the formation stage, members had difficulty assuming responsibility for the group and for making group decisions.

Did the structure provide for new learning, reinforcement of current level of functioning or adaptation, or did it reinforce functioning below current level of adaptation? Explain and give rationale.

Members were able to verbalize their individual concerns regarding managing life tasks on discharge. By being encouraged to share these concerns, members began to talk about what they wanted rather than what their family and friends wanted.

Did the structure provide an opportunity for evaluation and feedback regarding the group procedures and member progress? Explain.

Yes. Members were actively encouraged to give the leaders feedback.

D. What changes would you make regarding group goals and structure for the next session, or if you were to lead this session again?

Use a more individual-centered activity, with the specific aim of goal setting.

E. Were you adequately prepared for the session? (Give rationale, considering such things as time, place, materials, and physical and emotional environment.)

I was not prepared for the degree to which members wanted to talk about their fears.

F. How did you function as leader? How did your behavior and role affect the group? Were you effective? (Give rationale.) What did you learn about yourself as group leader?

I learned that although the value of the group is apparent to me, members need time to learn the value it has for them. Hence, a group decision-making task was too premature for this stage of the group.

G. Was the group interaction as you anticipated? If problems occurred, what processes can you identify as a basis for understanding the problems?

I expected more group problem solving and group-centered support than was realistic. Member trust and more group experience are necessary to achieve those ends.

H. In the future, what might you do differently as group leader? (Give rationale.)

I would assume a more active role in structuring an individual task for group members and assume more of the group maintenance roles.

CASE STUDY NUMBER 3
Community-Based Occupational Therapy Group

A Senior Activity Group in the Formation Stage

Group Session Plan Protocol

A. Name of Group   Activity Group

Date   August 16, fourth session out of ten

B. Specific goals for the group session
To increase interaction between members
To actively participate in group activities
To enjoy the group experience

C. Specific goals for group members if different from those just listed and goals for each group member
For Sophie, who is often confused, to show less confusion when attempting a task.
For Agnes, to attend and remain involved in the activity for the entire meeting.
For Tom, to ask for assistance when needed.

D. Description of and rationale for methods and procedures
1. Provide members with a group-centered activity where each group member can contribute to the total finished task. Show a collage made of the same materials as a model so that members can have a clear idea of what their finished product might look like.
2. Provide an activity that adapts comfortably to the different skills levels of individual members. The materials for making the collage range from applying stickers to cut and paste pictures from magazines. Also, members are to be encouraged to ask for help from other group members should they need help.
3. Decrease sense of isolation by building group cohesiveness.

E. Description of and rationale for leadership role
   1. Support and promote group discussion and interaction.
   2. Help members understand the purpose of the group's activity.
   3. Provide cueing as needed.
   4. To instill feelings of safety and belonging.

F. Describe necessary preparations
   Review session plan with aide.
   Gather supplies necessary for group activity including model collage.
   Prepare members for group activity by reminding them of the activity planning they had at the end of the last group session. Remind them of the group decision that the finished collage would be posted on the wall of the activity room for the Senior Center Open House next week.

G. List material and equipment needed:
   • Large construction paper of several colors so that group members can choose the color they like.
   • Magazines, precut magazine pictures, stickers, color pencils, glue and scissors.
   • Model of collage.

H. Time and sequence outline for sessions, including what you will do and say as leader and what the group will do; consider both content and process.
   1. Greetings and member distribution of name tags (approximately 10 minutes).
   2. Introduction to group activity, purpose, goals, and methods with visual cueing. Show model of group collage and point out how different materials were used. Remind members of the group decision made at the last meeting that the group collage would be posted on the wall of the activity room for the Senior Center Open House next week (approximately 15 minutes).
   3. Members choose color of large construction paper for their collage (approximately 5 minutes).
   4. Members make collage with assistance of leader and aide with adaptation as necessary. Leader assumes task and maintenance roles if needed. Members are encouraged to help each other and to ask for help as needed (approximately 40 minutes).
   5. Bring closure to the activity. Encourage members to share their experience in doing this activity. Also encourage members to share their degree of satisfaction or dissatisfaction with the collage and/or with the collage process. Help volunteering member to attach collage to the wall.

I. Other information pertinent to this specific session:
   For example: Will there be any new members, coleaders, or guests? Is

there an unusual tone on the unit or special event that is about to occur
or just occurred for the individual member or group?

Yes, John will be absent. Should members inquire about whether to leave
space for John's contribution the leader will refer this decision to the
group.

Session Evaluation Form Protocol

A. **Name of Group**   Activity Group

   Date   August 16

B. **Were the goals accomplished? (Give rationale and state outcome.)**

   1. **Member interaction:**   Members shared materials and there was discussion about where to place individual contributions on the collage.
   Some members expressed their opinions regarding the activity and
   gave each other feedback.

   Group-centered activity: The activity was the idea of a group participant and all members agreed to this choice of activity. Leader was supportive of the group's ability to carry out the task by providing needed
   materials and guidance. Some members needed cueing to get started but
   all participated to the level of their ability.

   Some members showed enjoyment of this activity by smiling and a few
   expressed satisfaction over the finished collage.

   2. **Was the session helpful in accomplishing short-term and long-term
   group and individual member goals?**
   Yes.

   Agnes stayed in the room during the entire session. This is the first time
   she has been able to do so. She participated in the activity for the entire
   meeting.

   Tom did ask Betty to cut out a picture from a magazine for him. He also
   asked her for approval as to where to glue the picture on the collage.

   Sophie was less confused about the task. She kept looking at the model
   as she decided what to contribute to the collage. It seemed to present a
   concrete guide for her.

   Betty responded to Tom's request for help and gave him the reassurance
   that he seemed to need.

   Clara asked if someone should put a picture in for John since he is a member of the group. The leader referred this decision to the group and the
   decision was made for someone to include John in the collage. Clara vol-
   unteered to do so.

   3. **Do you have any evidence that the sessions have been helpful to the
   members' functioning outside of the group?   Not yet.**

C. Was the group structure adequate for accomplishing the goals? Give rationale and consider: leadership; time/length of meeting; open vs. closed
   group; time, sequence, methods and procedures; media/modalities/tech-

niques employed; norms/behaviors reinforced implicitly or explicitly; methods of reinforcement; and stage of group's development.

1. A closed group format was needed for members to get to know each other. Socialization was an important goal of this group.
2. The time/length of this group was adequate for accomplishing goals. Time was needed for the members to greet each other, to remember their names as well as to orient themselves to the general surroundings. Time was needed to review the decisions made at the previous meeting for members who often experience memory loss.
3. The sequence, methods and procedures for the activity were well established. A model of a finished collage using the same materials was presented and described in detail to help clarify the activity goal. The concept of a collage as a group product was emphasized.
4. Members are still in the forming stage of group development.

Did the structure prove optimal "action" or "flow activity" for a "flow state" to occur?
The flow state was slow in starting but eventually all members became involved in the activity.

Did the structure provide optimal purposeful, self-initiated, spontaneous, and group-centered "action" for cognitive and emotional impact, skill learning, and adaptation to occur through "occupation"?
The activity was self initiated by a group member; it was also purposeful (to make a collage to put on the wall for the Open House). It did involve spontaneous action (choices of color of background and placement of items on the collage). Group action was demonstrated by a number of members.

Did the structure provide for new learning or reinforcement of current level of functioning or adaptation, or did it reinforce functioning below current level of adaptation? Explain and give rationale.
The structure of the activity promoted reinforcement of previously learned skills while contributing to the current level of functioning of the members. It enabled members to participate at a parallel through cooperative level. The activity helped to reinforce life roles of the past or present, such as the role of help giver and supporter or the role of one seeking help. Also, Clara did take steps to have John included as a group member contributing to the group collage thus acknowledging a sense of the group members being a group rather than a collection of individuals.

Did the structure provide an opportunity for evaluation and feedback regarding the group procedures and member progress? Explain.
Leader and aide provided ongoing positive feedback to members regarding both their efforts and productivity. Some feedback was directed to individuals and some to the group as a whole. A separate processing period was included in the design of the session to get direct feedback from the members regarding this activity and the group's progress, thus pro-

viding further reflection and processing of group events and experiences. Leader was able to observe member reactions and comments to the various parts of the task.

D. What changes would you make in group goals and structure for the next session, or if you were to lead this session again?

If I were to redo this session I would make the following changes:

1. I would pencil in a circle or oval on the construction board where the collage materials were to be pasted thus providing more structure for the members in this step of the task. This was a difficult step for them in the "flow" of the activity.

2. Leafing through the magazines provided a distraction for some members, so I would pre-cut pages from magazines and add them to available materials.

3. I would provide dampened paper towels for wiping sticky fingers after gluing.

E. Were you adequately prepared for the session? (Give rationale, considering such things as time, place, materials, and physical and emotional environment.)

Yes. Given that this was the fourth session of the group we were well aware of the needs for structure of the group in undertaking a group-centered activity.

F. How did you function as leader? How did your behavior and role affect the group? Were you effective? (Give rationale.) What did you learn about yourself as group leader?

We functioned effectively as group leaders during this session. We were attentive to cues from group members and used those cues to direct or redirect the group and particular members. As leader and assistant we had carefully discussed how we could work together in this group. We found that modeling cooperative behavior encouraged members to help each other. The assistant took the role of being primarily involved with the task of the group while the leader focused primarily on the maintenance functions. Although we had planned well for the group session, we learned the importance of being flexible within the structure and following the group's lead thus supporting self-initiated and group-centered action.

G. Was the group interaction as you anticipated? If problems occurred, what processes can you identify as a basis for understanding the problems?

Not exactly. We did not anticipate Clara's concern about including the absent member in the group collage. This created a presence of group solidarity not previously manifested and contributed to the group being more cohesive and cooperative, on the whole, than in previous sessions.

H. In the future, what might you do differently as group leader? (Give rationale.)

I would be willing to take greater risk with the complexity of the task. However with this group, I need to keep the activities positive and allow members to feel competent. This may mean that some members may not be encouraged to be as creative as they might be at this stage of group development.

Review Questions

1. When does the formation stage begin in a group and what are the characteristics of this stage?
2. What types of information might a leader include in his or her introductory statement to the group?
3. What are the two primary issues of the formation stages of a group?
4. What kinds of group-centered actions might be expected at this stage of group development?
5. What does "setting the climate," mean?
6. One of the roles of the leader is to teach members to assume responsibility for themselves in the group. How might a leader accomplish this task?
7. How does the structure of the group session influence the amount and type of member participation in the group?

References

Berne, E. (1963). The Structure and Dynamics of Organizations and Groups. New York: Grove Press.

Bradford, L. P. (1978). Group Formation and Development. In L. P. Bradford (ed.), Group Development (2nd ed.). La Jolla, CA: University Associates, pp. 4–12.

Corey, G., and Corey, M. S. (1982). Groups: Process and Practice (2nd ed.). Monterey, CA: Brooks/Cole.

Gibb, J., and Gibb, L. (1967). Humanistic elements in group growth. In J. Bugenthal (ed.), Challenges of Humanistic Psychology. New York: McGraw-Hill.

Napier, R. K., and Gershenfeld, M. K. (1983). Making Groups Work: A Guide for Group Leaders. Boston: Houghton Mifflin.

Rogers, C. (1969). Freedom to Learn. Columbus, OH: Merrill.

Rogers, C. (1970). Carl Rogers on Encounter Groups. New York: Harper & Row.

Truax, C., and Mitchell, K. (1971). Research on certain therapist intrapersonal skills in relation to process and outcome. In A. Bergin and S. Garfield (eds.), Handbook of Psychotherapy and Behavior Change. New York: John Wiley & Sons.

Yalom, I. D. (1975). The Theory and Practice of Group Psychotherapy (2nd ed.). New York: Basic Books, p. 120.

Yalom, I. D. (1983). Inpatient Group Psychotherapy. New York: Basic Books.

Chapter **8**
Stage Three: Development

Individuals are unique; therefore, one can rightfully expect that patterns in the development of a group will vary from group to group. Nevertheless, all groups demonstrate certain features. We have explored this principle in our examination of the aspects common to the formation stage. In this chapter, we describe the features characteristic of the group's development stage. More specifically, this chapter emphasizes leadership issues and individual and group expectations. The topics of assessing progress and identifying and managing problems will be discussed in the context of the group's action in the development stage. The leader's functions and intervention strategies in the development stage will be explained. These functions include involving members in setting goals, adapting the task to the stage of the group and individual members, and encouraging group member roles. Again, we will apply these concepts to the two case studies.

Issues and Expectations

The life of a group is multidimensional. At a concrete level, the functional group is composed of individuals, an activity, and a physical environment. At a symbolic level, the group has a purpose, both implicit and explicit, a set of dynamics and processes, and internal and external motivational forces. All of these factors are interacting at any given moment. In a sense these factors define the group's "metaspace," which is not something one can stop in time. The metaspace is an experience of the moment. Neutral observers and group members could probably describe the group in similar ways, yet it is likely each would also experience it a bit differently. Hence, the concrete and symbolic levels of a group are not readily distinguishable.

The purpose of the group is health and adaptation for its members. To accomplish this purpose, the leader strives to create an environment conducive to purposeful, self-initiated, spontaneous, and group-centered action. Because groups progress through stages with unique characteristics (Cohen and Smith, 1976; Corey and Corey, 1982; Garland and Frey, 1970; Garland, Jones, and Kolodny, 1973; Klein, 1972), the leader must use a variety of strategies. Thus, the leadership functions in the development stage may vary a great deal. Our intent is to suggest a general scheme for assessing the group's ongoing progress and identifying and managing problems. Certain issues are typical of this stage, and each can be met with appropriate responses (see Table 8-1).

Assessing Progress

To assess the group's progress, we suggest that the leader and, whenever possible, the group, attempt to identify problems at the concrete and symbolic levels. Such a review might occur at the beginning of a meeting, at the end of a session, at the completion of a task, or intermittently during the session. Some therapists prefer to designate a period for evaluating the session, such as the final 10 minutes. Other leaders might feel that this sort of strict scheduling breaks the flow of action or activity (Box 8-1). The timing will depend ultimately on the individual leader's style and the group members' attention span, ability to delay gratification, need for closure, and immediacy of the problem. Regardless of these considerations, in every instance, the leader must evaluate the group and individual members' progress.

Structured and unstructured observation methods are used to assess the group's ongoing progress. Structured methods provide the leader and members specific formats for systematically noting and recording behavior, events, and reactions. In addition to the methods suggested in Chapter 5 (see Figs. 5-2 through 5-6), the members or the leader may choose to design observation formats specifically suited to the group's needs. In contrast, unstructured observation methods require the leader or members to examine progress by spontaneously analyzing the group's process and dynamics. Miles (1981) suggests two techniques for the study of group behavior particularly relevant to the functional group in the development stage: "trainer process comments" (p. 115) and "intermittent process analysis" (p. 117). "Trainer [or leader] comments (a) illuminate the immediate problems facing the group, and (b) help build in the process-analysis function as a central feature of the group's work structure" (p. 115). Miles (1981) suggests that once the group has some experience with

Table 8-1
Group Membership Needs Related to Action: Development Stage

Development Stage Issues*	Purposeful Action	Self-Initiated Action	Spontaneous (Here-and-Now) Action	Group-Centered Action	Leader Skills Employed
Concern over acceptance or rejection as result of change Testing the safety of the group	Goals and structure Minimal risk in task Clear and consistent rules, limits, expectations, and routines Protection from attack	Encouragement and support for exploratory behavior	Encouragement and support for initiative taken in group and expression of thoughts and feelings in here and now As action occurs, group-centered leadership encouragement Modeling of group task and maintenance roles	Explicit group norms Recognition and clarification of stage issue in context of dependence versus independence theme Clarification of reality	Genuineness and empathy Listening and responding Concreteness Reality testing Group task analysis and adaptation
Struggle between safety and involvement	Clear options and alternatives	Encouragement for task involvement and expression of positive and negative reactions and feelings		Encouragement for cohesive member sharing of task roles Leader input as needed by group Recognition and clarification of stage issue in context of intimacy theme concerning passivity versus activity or personal versus group wishes and needs	Modeling behavior Self-disclosure Feedback
Control and power struggles	Consistency and safety of	Permissive environment		Flexibility in assuming leadership	Confrontation

continued

Table 8-1
Group Membership Needs Related to Action:
Development Stage (*Continued*)

Development Stage Issues*	Purposeful Action	Self-Initiated Action	Spontaneous (Here-and-Now) Action	Group-Centered Action	Leader Skills Employed
(conflict) with leader and other members	individuals Support and encouragement for member leadership Task appears useful to each individual	Opportunity for action matches individual member abilities		and social-emotional roles as able Support and encouragement for member leadership Recognition and clarification of stage issue in context of dependency versus counter-dependency needs or ambivalence regarding autonomy theme	

*Corey, G., and Corey, M. S. Groups: Process and Practice (2nd ed.), p. 194. Copyright 1977, 1982 by Wadsworth, Inc. Reprinted by permission of Brooks/Cole Publishing Co., Monterey, CA.

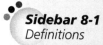

Sidebar 8-1
Definitions

Trainer process comments: *Leader's observations that illuminate the group's immediate problems.*

Intermittent process analysis: *Ongoing questioning by group members as to what is happening in the group and why, as well as how group behavior can change for the better.*

Box 8-1
Act Promptly

We suggest that issues or problems be addressed as they occur in the group.

---

trainer process comments, the group can establish that members should spontaneously comment on what is happening. "In effect, group members are continually asking, 'What is happening? What is making these things happen? How can we change our behavior for the better?'" (p. 117).

If the members are encouraged to be evaluators and observers to determine the validity of leader assessment, the methods should yield data pertaining to the group's outcomes and operation at the symbolic and concrete levels. The information gathered concerns members' actual functioning in the group environment and reports of behavior outside the group. Two questions guide the assessment: "As a result of the group's interaction, are members learning the skills and occupational behaviors necessary for adaptation, and are they better able to fulfill their health needs?" and "Is the group's structure, process, and content conducive to appropriate action in the development stage?" (See Table 8-1).

Identifying and Managing Problems

In the development stage, one may expect problems that are characteristic of group members learning to work on a mutual task. Problems may derive from the group as a whole or from individual members. In attempting to identify the group's needs, the leader must ask a basic question: "What is inhibiting the group's movement toward purposeful, self-initiated, spontaneous, group-centered action?" The leader must examine every aspect of the functional group to answer this question.

Bradford, Stock, and Horwitz (1978) mention some of the more common group problems (Box 8-2). These include "conflict or fight," "apathy and nonparticipation," and "inadequate decision making" (p. 63). They also suggest specific origins for these group problems. Members who demonstrate fight behavior may view the group and themselves in one of four possible ways. They may feel "frustrated because they feel unable to meet the demands made of them" (p. 63). Their main goal may be "to find status in the group" (p. 64) rather than follow the goals or task set by the leader or other members. The members may feel a greater loyalty to "outside groups of conflicting interests" (p. 64). Finally, the members may "feel involved and are working hard on a problem" (p. 64) and therefore resent the disruption or conflict from others. Members may respond with apathy if "the problem upon which the group is working does not seem important to the members, or . . . [seems] less important than some other problem on which they would prefer to be working. . . . [Or] the problem may seem important to members, but there are reasons which lead them to avoid attempting to solve the problem" (p. 67). Members also respond with apathy

---

> Box 8-2
> **Problems that Arise**
>
> Common group problems in the development stage include the following:
>
> - **Conflict or fight**
> - **Apathy and nonparticipation**
> - **Indequate decision making**

---

when a group has "inadequate procedures for solving the problem" (p. 68). Related to this is the feeling that members are "powerless about influencing final decisions" (p. 68). Finally, "A prolonged and deep fight among a few members . . . [may have] dominated the group" (p. 68), leaving others to feel apathetic.

Inadequate decision making may result from unsatisfactory group interactions. For example, "there has been premature calling for a decision, or the decision is too difficult, or the group is low in cohesiveness and lacks faith in itself" or again "the decision area may be threatening to the group, either because of unclear consequences, fear of reaction of other groups, or fear of failure for the individuals" (p. 72).

In addition to the group's difficulties with task and maintenance functions, individual members may have problems. A group member may lack the skills or experience necessary to accomplish his or her role or function in the group. A group member may also have unrealistic notions regarding his or her skills or ability to complete the task. In discussing action, Csikszentmihalyi (1975) points out that "perhaps the most salient element of the flow state is a sense of control over the environment. A person has to feel that his ability to act is adequate to meet the opportunities for action available. 'Inner' skills and 'outer' challenges must be in balance before the flow state can be experienced" (p. 191).

The problems of individual members vary, and the leader should consider the following problem areas when trying to identify specific problems:

1. Lack of opportunity for skill practice and modeling
2. Inadequate positive reinforcement
3. Secret or conflicting goals
4. Inadequate information
5. Ill-formed defense mechanisms
6. Poor self-esteem
7. Lack of task skills or social interaction skills
8. Physical, neuromotor, or cognitive limits to functioning
9. Overappraisal or underappraisal of skills
10. Overappraisal or underappraisal of environmental demands

Problems can also arise on the symbolic level; problems in the group's structure and processes can inhibit a group's development. Although we assume that group leaders have positive intentions, they may lack group leadership skills or be unaware of the ways in which they are fostering group problems. Some of the problems often stemming from group leadership are as follows:

- The activity is not matched to the group's abilities, processes, goals, or environment.
- The activities fail to meet members' interests or basic needs (safety, approval, self-esteem).
- Group goals are unclear, unrealistic, or not understood.
- Emotional environment does not support the group's efforts or those of individual members.
- Group members lack the necessary skills to perform a specific task.
- The leader is unaware of secret or conflicting goals because of mechanisms for receiving feedback communication.
- The physical climate is not conducive to achieving the group's purpose. (The room is too hot or too small; the group is too big for everyone to be heard or understood.)
- The composition of the group does not allow for cohesiveness.
- Members are neither encouraged to contribute to the goals of the group or to the group procedures, nor to help each other directly.
- The leader does not encourage the group to evaluate its procedures, process, and effectiveness. This may include prematurely summarizing group themes, actions, and communication, both verbal and nonverbal.
- The distribution of leadership and membership roles is inadequate.
- Group members are not given the opportunity to test ideas and possible courses of action.
- The leader does not establish clear limits and expectations or is passive in dealing with disruptive group behavior or interference from outside the group.
- The leader shows favoritism to particular group members or to subgroups through nonverbal or verbal communication.

If a leader is concerned with his or her leadership style, this list can serve as a guide for self-examination, supervision, and identification of leadership problems. In some instances, solving a seemingly minor problem of the physical environment can eliminate apparent leadership problems. For example, if members feel they are not heard adequately, a change from a noisy room may create an environment in which leader and members are more relaxed and therefore can listen to each other more easily. An advantage of coleadership is that leaders can share the task of identifying problems. One leader might more naturally follow and address leadership problems at the concrete level of the group, and the other attend to problems at the symbolic level.

Leader Intervention Strategies

Many strategies can be used to intervene in the numerous problems just described. To influence the group's process and outcome, the leader can consciously alter the group's structure through three strategies: (1) involving members in setting goals, (2) adapting the task more closely to the group and individual members, and (3) encouraging group member roles. To use these methods, the leader should be familiar with the functional skills and strategies described in Chapter 5.

Involving Members in Setting Goals

An essential feature of occupational therapy is the patient's participation in his plan of treatment. As Yerxa (1967) candidly points out:

> Occupational therapy has been unique, historically, because of the client's participation in his own treatment. Choice has been so fundamental to our thinking that we have questioned whether procedures which are done to the person, over which he has no control, should be called occupational therapy. (p. 3)

A key leadership function in the group, therefore, is to enable the group members to become involved in establishing goals (Box 8-3). The strategy employed varies according to the individual's readiness, as well as the group's maturity or degree of social–emotional cohesiveness (Fig. 8-1).

The value of member involvement in goal setting should not be underestimated. In their study of making choices, Henry, Nelson, and Duncombe (1984) found that "subjects who were not permitted choices in completing the activity perceived themselves as less powerful only when they participated in the activity in the presence of others in the same situation" (p. 249). By encouraging the group members to make choices about the group's goals, the leader establishes a norm that supports the notion that the group will reinforce members' sense of control and mastery. Rather than creating a group culture or set of norms that instills a feeling of hopelessness, the leader aims to empower members by teaching, through experience or action, the value of achieving a personally selected goal. It appears likely, in light of the Henry, Nelson, and Duncombe (1984) study, that having a sense of choice is particularly important to individuals when an activity is conducted in a group setting.

Even if explicitly stated by the leader, group goals often seem ambiguous to the members in the initial phase of a group's development. In the case of a

---

Box 8-3
Leader Strategies

Strategies a leader can use to alter the group's course are as follows:

- **Goal-setting with group members**
- **Matching the task with the group and its members**
- **Encouraging group member roles**

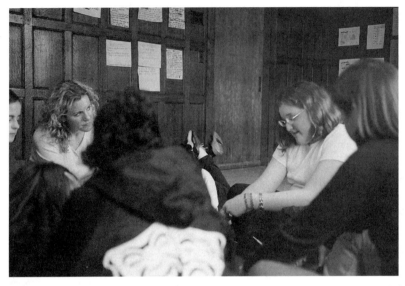

Figure 8-1. Member involvement in setting goals. (Photograph by Sarah Brezinsky.)

short-term group, with a limited time frame, the leader must rapidly focus members' attention and energy on goal setting. The many factors that influence the selection of goals by the group and individual members, as well as the recurring nature of goal selection during the group's course, make member involvement in goal setting an ongoing leadership task.

To understand the intervention strategy for involving members in goal selection, we should examine factors that can influence the formation of group goals. Cartwright and Zander (1968) have identified three factors that appear to influence "goal formation":

- Motives of members: These can be of a personal interest to individual members or solely in the best interests of the group.
- Superordinate group goals: These focus on long-term purposes and group objectives.
- The group and its social surroundings: This includes other groups that exert influence on the group's goals.

Research has also demonstrated that members will take greater risks and be more willing to work together toward the group's purpose if they are involved in making a group decision or specifying a group goal (Cartwright and Zander, 1968).

How can the leader instill hope and facilitate member involvement in goal setting? If the functional group is conducted within an institution or with some outside directives, the leader should first and always keep the members informed of the group's general purpose and resources. After giving general information on these factors, the leader should ask members what their needs are.

Leaders can also give member feedback and encourage the members to give each other feedback about the occupational behaviors displayed in the group and their adaptiveness. Members often find it useful to hear about the procedures and formats used in similar groups. Through these various strategies, the leader helps members and the group as a whole define its problems and needs.

Functional group members are often severely impaired in their ability to cognitively, emotionally, or socially impart information or formulate goals. Insecurity about performance skills, such as management of new prosthetic devices, can also contribute to difficulty in goal setting. Therefore, the leader, in the course of the group's development, must at times actively establish formats for goal setting. This can be accomplished by structuring various activities to help members clarify their goals, actively listening to members and reflecting back what is being said or not said in concrete terms, observing members and reporting back what is being done or not done, and encouraging group members to report back to the group their experiences outside the group as pertinent to the here-and-now action in the group.

Finally, through their verbal and nonverbal behavior, leaders must demonstrate that every member's opinion is important to the group's functioning. Similarly, the leader must be aware of members' changing needs and the necessity for involving members in goal setting throughout the course of the group's development.

Task Adaptation

The development stage builds on the formation stage of the group. In the first stage a group climate is established, group goals and roles are clarified, and the basis for trusting relationships is formed (Box 8-4). The development stage includes what Corey and Corey (1982) call the "transition stage" and "working stage" of a group. They point out that "the transitional phase of a group's development is marked by feelings of anxiety and defenses in the form of various resistances" (p. 194). In the functional group, certain member behaviors or "resistances" might appear: concern over group acceptance or rejection if members change, testing the safety of the group, a struggle between safety and involvement, and control and power struggles or conflicts with the leader or with the other group members (p. 194). After the group has worked out these issues, it passes into the working stage of a group. Members are able to function as

Box 8-4
Continually Adapting

As the group continues to develop, the leader must adapt the task and his or her strategies to meet the newly evolved needs of the group.

a cohesive unit; there is open communication; the leadership functions are shared; and members feel there is hope for change (pp. 195–196). Interestingly, beginning group leaders commonly feel that they have done something wrong when developmental problems arise in a group. We believe these problems are characteristic of groups learning to act together on a task and that for the group to progress, it must work through the issues specific to the development stage.

A group leader can use specific strategies in adapting the group's task structure and process in the development stage. First, the leader should identify the dominant characteristic displayed by group members. Second, the leader then grades or structures the activity to allow the group to learn how to work out the issue. For example, a leader might notice that members are late for a group meeting and do not bring the supplies necessary to complete a planned activity. By confronting the group with empathy, the leader can begin to clarify if a power struggle exists. Perhaps the leader learns that members felt the leader or a subgroup of members imposed the activity choice on them. In this instance, the group can be supportively encouraged to examine alternative ways to approach the decision-making process. The leader might suggest that the group role-play confronting an authority figure or practice ways to offer an opinion or give information. Ultimately, the leader is permitting a safe rebellion and teaching new behavior or adaptive skills by being accepting, yet protecting, the safety of the group.

If the group is an open group, one can expect that issues will recur as the membership of the group changes. Similarly, if the membership is heavily weighted with individuals who are experiencing difficulty with a particular problem—such as separation problems of adolescence—one should expect that problem to be reflected in the type of group development issue that arises. For example, power and control struggle relative to the leadership or task might become problematic. In a closed group, the leader has an advantage in being able to process the group's actions and plan strategies on a session-to-session basis. Finally, given the nature of a short-term, open group, of which there are many in acute care settings, the functional group leader must view the group's development and plan for it because all of it might exist in one session. Thus, one session might include issues concerning the formation, development, and termination stages. For example, the tone on a psychiatric inpatient unit might be rapidly assessed before the group meeting and an activity suggested to the group based on the formulation (Box 8-5).

Box 8-5
Need for Structure

The therapist working in an acute care setting will need to be more prescriptive or restrictive in adapting activities than would the leader working in a long-term setting.

Encouraging Group Member Roles

For group members to be encouraged to assume the various group membership and leadership roles, they must be involved in planning the group and assuming responsibility for action in accordance with the group's stage of development. First, members must be taught the skills necessary to engage in a group task. Such skills as giving feedback, receiving feedback, reality testing, speaking in the present tense, decision making, and assessing progress can be modeled by the group leader or leaders and practiced by the members.

Once the group members have the prerequisite skills, the leader can encourage members to assume the task and maintenance functions of the group through the following techniques:

- Involve all group members in defining the group's purpose, procedures, and norms and in observing the group's behavior.
- Positively reinforce members' strengths, compensate for deficits through structuring the group's task at levels members can manage, and avoid focusing on members' limitations.
- Provide the group with the resources necessary for task completion, that is, an appropriate room and access to needed materials.
- Act as a resource person and facilitator rather than an authority or rescuer.
- Use a coleader, if possible, to model ways to share responsibility and give support. In other words, do not look to the group for emotional support or supervision. Members should feel that the leader or leaders are present to enable the group to achieve positive action rather than to meet the leader's needs.
- Provide some structure but do not overwhelm the group so that members feel useless or not understood. Too much structure fosters dependency and stifles self-initiated action.
- Sanction testing a variety of behaviors within the limit of the group's safety.
- Help members to assess realistically the consequences of their actions and the relationship between behavior in the group and behavior outside the group.

Leader Emotional Response

The development stage of a group presents special challenges to leaders with a high need for control and being perceived as an authority. As the group becomes more cohesive members will have less of a need to perceive the leader as all knowing. In developing stronger bonds, members will struggle with each other and the leader for power and control. Acting out behaviors such as lateness and unexplained absences test the group's limits and stability. Although these reactions can be expected, they can cause strong emotional reactions in leaders as well as members.

Coleaders can help each other to monitor reactions that are counterproductive to the group. They may find disruptions in their working relationship that mirror struggles in the group such as vying for control, favoritism, and so on. Monitoring such acting out on the leader's part is paramount to the group's survival in the development stage. Self-reflective questions (Box 8-6) can help

---

Box 8-6
Leader Self-Reflective Questions

In the development stage, leaders often ask themselves self-reflective questions such as:

1. In the past, how have I dealt with conflict in a group situation? What is my reaction to the group becoming more cohesive and members assuming more authority over their own process and procedures?

2. Have there been unusual behaviors in the group such as premature loss of members, absences, or lateness? What is my reaction? What strategies have I used to manage these boundary violations? What conflicts may the group be experiencing to lead to such behaviors? How can I support and guide the group at this point is its development?

3. Have I or my coleader, if any, been acting differently toward each other in or outside of the group? Are these actions helpful to the group's and individual member's development? Are there feelings growing that have not been discussed or unresolved conflicts at the root of the turmoil? For example, do I feel unusually competitive with my coleader? Does this resonate with unresolved sibling rivalry left from my own primary family relationships or from an adult partnership?

---

leaders to self-examine their emotional responses and to identify patterns in their own reactions to working in the development stage (see Case Studies 1, 2, and 3, Session Evaluation Form Protocols).

Conclusion

Just as the formation stage, the development stage has particular issues and problems requiring specific responses by leaders. The issues that arise are part of the growth critical to the well-being of the group and its ultimate success regarding certain goals. In the following, the various features and concerns of the development stage are illustrated in the group session plans and session evaluation forms completed for both groups in the case studies.

CASE STUDY NUMBER 1
Open Occupational Therapy Group

Integrating the New Member in the Development Stage

Group Session Plan Protocol

A. Name of group   Project Group

Date   June 13

B. Specific goals for the group session

To experience success in an interdependent task.

To express feelings and thoughts in the present tense.

To express positive and negative reactions and feelings.

C. Specific goals for group members if different from those just listed and goals for each group member

Mary (new member): Integrate into group.

Other group members: Express negative and positive feelings about having a new group member.

D. Description of and rationale for methods and procedures

Summarize previous session (to reinforce learning for "old" members and to integrate new member).

Decide on theme and group procedures for painting group mural (to provide an opportunity for expressing and processing threatening feelings regarding having a new member in the group; activity is familiar to old members and provides a role for all members; there is no one correct way to paint a mural, hence, no opportunity for failure).

E. Description of and rationale for leadership role

Encourage members to talk about their fears and anger regarding perceived potential loss of attention in group and own anxieties when entering a new group.

Rationale: Provides group an opportunity to reality test expectations of leader and group; recognizes stage issue of dependence versus independence and at the same time reinforces that it is safe to express feelings in the group; frees the group's energy for spontaneous, purposeful, group-centered action; and clarifies how individual and group dynamics can affect decision making and action.

F. Describe necessary preparations

Review and discuss plan among group leaders.

Prepare new member for group in a pregroup interview: Discuss recent activities of group, its goals, and norms. Reinforce notion that new members are encouraged to participate at their own pace and that it is likely that she will feel somewhat confused, perhaps like an outsider, until she has some experience with the group's procedures and processes.

Cut paper and gather necessary supplies.

G. List material and equipment needed

Poster paints in the primary colors

Ten wide paint brushes

Paper cups, water, and tape

Large roll of paper for mural

H. Time and sequence outline for session, including what you will say and do as the leader and what the group will do; consider both content and process

Introduction of new and old members; review of group's purpose and procedures (approximately 5 minutes).

Review previous group session with group input (approximately 5 minutes).

Plan group mural, encouraging group member roles (approximately 10 minutes).

Members paint mural (approximately 15 minutes).

Process session and plan next session—see leadership role (approximately 10 minutes).

I. Other information pertinent to this specific session

For example: Will there be any new members, coleaders, or guests? Is there an unusual tone on the unit or special event that is about to occur or just occurred for the individual member or group?

There is a new female member joining the group.

This session will take place on a Friday, and the group will not meet again until Monday.

A highly esteemed group member was discharged yesterday.

Session Evaluation Form Protocol

A. Name of Group   Project Group

Date   June 13

B. Were the goals accomplished? (Give rationale and state outcome.)

Yes. All group members participated in the painting of a mural.

The theme selected was "Birth and Death." Members shared positive feelings and negative reactions about the group with the new member.

Was the session helpful in accomplishing short-term and long-term group and individual member goals?
Yes.

Do you have any evidence that the session(s) have been helpful to the members' functioning (adaptation) outside of the group?

Partially. In the community meeting after this group session, some members discussed the need for a unit orientation brochure.

C. Was the group structure adequate for accomplishing the goals? Give rationale and consider: leadership; time/length of meeting; open versus closed group; time, sequence, methods and procedures; media/modalities/techniques employed; norms/behaviors reinforced implicitly or explicitly; methods of reinforcement; and stage of group's development.

Yes. However, in the next session, it seems advisable to let the group members take a more active role in assuming the task roles.

Did the structure provide optimal "action" or "flow activity" for a "flow state" to occur?

Yes. By having the group members select a mural theme, they were challenged to express their feelings in an activity that matched their capabilities.

Did the structure provide optimal purposeful, self-initiated, spontaneous, and group-centered "action" for cognitive and emotional impact, skill learning, and adaptation to occur through "occupation"?

Yes. However, in the next session the group members should be encouraged to select an activity modality so that they can examine their decision-making process and tendency to rely on the group leaders.

Did the structure provide for new learning, reinforcement of current level of functioning or adaptation, or did it reinforce functioning below current level of adaptation? Explain and give rationale.

The structure did provide for new learning. Members learned that rather than heightening a sense of deprivation and isolation, expressing their thoughts and emotions enabled them to feel closer to other members and gratified by the group's efforts.

Did the structure provide an opportunity for evaluation and feedback regarding the group procedures and member progress? Explain.

Yes. Having a structured process time at the beginning and end of the session eased the new member's transition into the group and gave the old members the feeling they were all heard.

D. What changes would you make regarding group goals and structure for the next session, or if you were to lead this session again?

In the next session the leaders should gently encourage members to assume more of the group task roles. In adapting the leader roles members should be urged to make simple task decisions, then sequence a plan of action, and, finally, detect when a change in action is needed.

E. Were you adequately prepared for the session? (Give rationale, considering such things as time, place, materials, and physical and emotional environment.)

Yes. The meeting started on time, all the necessary materials were available, and the leaders provided a supportive, enthusiastic, and consistent environment.

F. How did you function as leader? How did your behavior and role affect the group? Were you effective? (Give rationale.) What did you learn about yourself as group leader?

I established the group's procedures for the session, encouraged members to participate in the task by asking for their opinions and feelings, and reality tested by exploring the relationship between member thoughts and feelings and behavior. I believe this was effective in bringing about a feeling of cohesiveness and safety in the group. Members became aware of similarities in their reactions. This should aid the members in assuming more responsibility for task roles and in testing out new role behaviors. I learned that it is more comfortable for me to explore member reactions when the group is involved in an expressive versus a constructive activity.

G. Was the group interaction as you anticipated? If problems occurred, what processes can you identify as a basis for understanding the problems?
As I anticipated, members relied heavily on the leaders for task structure and emotional support. Expressing negative and positive feelings is quite difficult for members, especially with a new member present. Given these issues, members' needs for leader approval and fear of loss of attention may have fostered the dependency.

H. In the future, what might you do differently as group leader? (Give rationale.)
In the future, to reinforce the idea of member choice and responsibility, I would suggest three alternative expressive art activities.

CASE STUDY NUMBER 2
Closed Occupational Therapy Group

Power and Control Relative to Leader and Task in the Development Stage

Group Session Plan Protocol

A. Name of Group   Energy Conservation/Time Management Group

 Date   fourth session out of eight—December 17

B. Specific goals for the group session
To learn energy-saving procedures, work simplification techniques, and organization of the environment to minimize energy output.

C. Specific goals for group members if different from those just listed and goals for each group member
Recognize ambivalence over dependency on leader, hospital, and significant others.

D. Description of and rationale for methods and procedures
Lecture, slide show, demonstration, practice, and discussion
Rationale: Audiovisuals will make procedures more concrete; discussion gives members an opportunity to vent feelings and get group support; and practice allows for some skill development.

E. Description of and rationale for leadership role
Teacher, encourager, supporter, and confronter
Rationale: To model techniques, reality test, and support members' emotional needs.

F. Describe necessary preparations.
Prepare audiovisuals, lecture, and work simulations.

G. List material and equipment needed.
Slides, screen, slide projector, and work simulation stations

H. Time and sequence outline for session, including what you will say and do as leader and what the group will do; consider both content and process.
Slide show and lecture
Group discussion
Practice techniques at work simulation stations

I. Other information pertinent to this specific session
For example: Will there be any new members, coleaders, or guests? Is there an unusual tone on the unit or special event that is about to occur or just occurred for the individual member or group?
Patients are preparing for hospital Christmas festivities.

Session Evaluation Form Protocol

A. Name of Group   Energy Conservation/Time Management Group

Date   December 17

B. Were the goals accomplished? (Give rationale and state outcome.)
Yes. Members were able to express concerns about being dependent on their families and their anger toward the therapist for not continuing the group after hospitalization. Members were able to demonstrate some procedures and techniques.

Was the session helpful in accomplishing short-term and long-term group and individual member goals?
Yes.

Do you have any evidence that the session(s) have been helpful to the members' functioning (adaptation) outside of the group?
Yes. Some members have requested the therapist give them written instructions to take home.

C. Was the group structure adequate for accomplishing the goals? Give rationale and consider: leadership; time/length of meeting; open versus closed group; time, sequence, methods and procedures; media/modalities/techniques employed; norms/behaviors reinforced implicitly or explicitly; methods of reinforcement; and stage of group's development.
Session should be expanded or group held more often. The pace seemed too quick and rushed.

Did the structure provide optimal "action" or "flow activity" for a "flow state" to occur?
No. More opportunity was needed for problem solving and practice.

Did the structure provide optimal purposeful, self-initiated, spontaneous, and group-centered "action" for cognitive and emotional impact, skill learning, and adaptation to occur through "occupation"?
No. More group problem solving and open-ended simulated problem situations would have been helpful for behavioral rehearsal.

Did the structure provide for new learning, reinforcement of current level of functioning or adaptation, or did it reinforce functioning below current level of adaptation? Explain and give rationale.
Yes. All members attempted to practice the techniques and discuss how the procedures would work or be problematic at home.

Did the structure provide an opportunity for evaluations and feedback regarding the group procedures and member progress? Explain.
Yes. The group discussion gave members an opportunity to give feedback and practice exercises and gave the leaders a chance to observe.

D. What changes would you make regarding group goals and structure for the next session, or if you were to lead this session again?
I would provide members with written materials illustrating and summarizing the techniques learned.

E. Were you adequately prepared for the session? (Give rationale, considering such things as time, place, materials, and physical and emotional environment.)
No. The goals were unrealistic and materials were needed.

F. How did you function as leader? How did your behavior and role affect the group? Were you effective? (Give rationale.) What did you learn about yourself as group leader?
Yes, I was effective in providing support through structure and room for group support to surface by pointing out common themes, issues, and alternative behaviors.

G. Was the group interaction as you anticipated? If problems occurred, what processes can you identify as a basis for understanding the problems?
The group members were somewhat more angry than I expected. This may be because of the upcoming holidays and related feelings regarding loss in functioning and impending discharge.

H. In the future, what might you do differently as group leader? (Give rationale.)
Divide group into pairs for practice session to increase member sharing and decrease dependence on leaders for instruction and support.

CASE STUDY NUMBER 3
Community-Based Occupational Therapy Group

Building Stronger Group Member Roles: An Activity Group for Seniors in the Development Stage

Group Session Plan Protocol

A. Name of Group   Activity Group

Date   August 30, sixth session out of ten.

B. Specific goals for the group session
To increase initiative in planning group activities.
To express feelings and thoughts in present tense (here and now).
To verbalize both positive and negative reactions to group activities.
To interact socially.
To experience enjoyment in self-expression.

C. Specific goals for group members if different from those mentioned already and goals for each group member
Sue and Betty were late for the group last week. If they are late again, to discuss this issue in the group.

D. Description of and rationale for methods and procedures
Summarize activity of previous session. Members decorated greeting cards. Clara observed that they had no verse written on the cards. Plan was made for group to write some poetry in this session.
With a collective poem, group members each contribute at least one line to a poem about a selected topic.
Rationale: Writing in a group allows elder participants to channel reminiscences and synthesize them into the poem. Poetry writing also encourages a deeper level of social interaction than previous group activities. The process of creating a collective poem validates everyone's experience and contribution.

E. Description of and rationale for leadership role
Support and encourage group discussion of positive and negative feelings about this activity.
Assist members in reminiscing process and in the selection of a topic for poem. Also, provide support for and acknowledge member contributions.
Provide structure for writing and repeating lines or phrases of the poem for those members who have auditory or visual deficits by reading each contribution aloud and writing it in large letters on newsprint.

F. Describe necessary preparations
Review and discuss session plan with aide.
Select examples of poems to read to the group.
Describe in detail the procedure for writing a group poem reassuring members that a contribution to the poem can be just a word, a phrase, or a line.

G. List material and equipment needed
Large newsprint paper, an easel stand and markers.
Pens and paper for members to record the poem(s) written by the group.

H. Time and sequence outline for sessions, including what you will do and say as leader and what the group will do; consider both content and process.

1. Greetings, distribution of nametags. Review group purposes and procedures (approximately 10 minutes).
2. Review of last session and group planning for today (approximately 10 minutes).
3. Introduce the activity of group poetry writing and the process of reminiscence of life events. Describe how a topic for the poem will be chosen from reminiscences. Read selected examples of poetry. Describe process of group poetry writing by having each member in turn, contribute a line, a word or a phrase to the poem (approximately 15 minutes).
4. Leader starts reminiscences by contributing a memory from childhood and asks group members to do likewise. As members come up with topics, the leader will record them on the newsprint and repeat them aloud. After approximately 20 minutes, the leader will read the list of topics and member will chose a topic for a poem.
5. As each group member makes a contribution to the poem, the leader will write it down on newsprint and read it aloud for all to hear. The member will be given a chance to change any word. Gentle prompting by the leader will help to ensure that members have satisfactorily expressed themselves before the next member will have his or her turn to add to the poem. The group will continue to go around in a circle so that all group members have the opportunity to participate and contribute to the collective poem (approximately 20 minutes)
6. The completed poem(s) will then be read aloud in its entirety and copied.
7. Ask members to share how they felt about today's activity and group experience (approximately 15 minutes).
8. For next week: Make a copy of poem for the group members to keep.

I. Other information pertinent to this specific session: For example: Will there be any new members, coleaders, or guests? Is there an unusual tone on the unit or special event that is about to occur or just occurred for the individual member or group?
No known event.

Session Evaluation Form Protocol

A. Name of Group   Activity Group

Date   August 30

B. Were the goals accomplished? (Give rationale and state outcome.)
Yes, partially. The reminiscence experience did not encourage the expression of thoughts and feelings in the "here and now"; however, members did express feelings about the activity in the "here and now" discussion at the end of the session. All members participated in the activity but Tom, Betty, and Sue said that they didn't really enjoy it. They were encouraged to take a more active role in the planning of activities in the future.

Was the session helpful in accomplishing short-term and long-term group and individual member goals?
Yes.

Do you have any evidence that the session(s) have been helpful to the members' functioning (adaptation) outside of the group?
Yes, partially. Some members do meet for coffee or lunch together before or after the group.

c. Was the group structure adequate for accomplishing the goals? Give rationale, and consider the following: leadership; time/length of meeting; open versus closed group; time, sequence, methods and procedures; media/modalities/techniques employed; norms/behaviors reinforced implicitly or explicitly; methods of reinforcement; and stage of group's development.
Yes. However, some members were only superficially involved in the poetry writing. One member stated that she never could write poetry. All members of the group did get involved in the reminiscence part of the activity, owing in part to the group norm that all group members participate in the activity at some level. This norm has been reinforced by group leader and some members, as well.

Did the structure provide optimal "action" or "flow activity" for a "flow state" to occur?
Yes. Particularly in the reminiscence part of the activity. Some members found it difficult to stop this part of the activity and proceed to the next part of writing the poem.

Did the structure provide optimal purposeful, self-initiated, spontaneous, and group-centered "action" for cognitive and emotional impact, skill learning, and adaptation to occur through "occupation"?
Yes. However, more progress needs to be made. Members need to be more involved in the activity selection and particularly in making the decisions needed to better adapt the activity to meet the particular needs of the group. These types of decisions are now primarily decided by the leader.

Did the structure provide for new learning or reinforcement of current level of functioning or adaptation, or did it reinforce functioning below current level of adaptation? Explain and give rationale.
Yes, the structure did provide for an expression of positive and negative feelings about the group activity. Some members did learn that their opinions were respected and welcomed and that they could influence the group planning process and thereby increase the degree of group satisfaction.

Did the structure provide an opportunity for evaluation and feedback regarding the group procedures and member progress? Explain.
Yes. The structured processing time at both the beginning and the end of the session assisted member involvement in the group's process.

D. What changes would you make regarding group goals and structure for the next session or if you were to lead this session again?

The leader should reassure members that their contributions to the group task are welcome and supported. Also, that they do possess the necessary skills to complete the task successfully and that they can ask for help from other members. Frail elderly members frequently hesitate to test skills that they may not have used recently.

E. Were you adequately prepared for the session? (Give rationale, considering such things as time, place, materials, and physical and emotional environment.)

Yes. The meeting started on time and leader and aide were prepared, materials at hand, and there was a supportive and consistent emotional environment.

F. How did you function as leader? How did your behavior and role affect the group? Were you effective? (Give rationale.) What did you learn about yourself as group leader?

The usual procedure for starting the group session was followed: A member gave each person (including leader and aide) their name tag. The leader greeted everyone and asked if any important events had happened since our last meeting. A review of the last session followed (including the process of selecting the activity for today). Additional comments or corrections were encouraged. This opening part of the group session seems to be effective in creating a mutually helping and safe, caring environment, creating a feeling of group cohesiveness. Some members seem to require time to readjust to the environment and climate of the group. I want to allow time for that to happen before starting the group activity, especially today because the group will be involved in an expressive rather than a constructive activity. I have learned to try to sense the pace of the group members and adjust my pace accordingly and to allow time for this in planning the session. At the end of the session, enough time remained for the members to share their observations and feelings without being hurried.

G. Was the group interaction as you anticipated? If problems occurred, what processes can you identify as a basis for understanding the problems?

Some members were more outspoken about their dislike of the activity than I had anticipated. I felt that creativity was a difficult and uncomfortable process for them and I encouraged them to become more involved in the discussion of activity selection, that everyone has likes and dislikes, and that I encourage them to share these with the group.

H. In the future, what might you do differently as group leader? (Give rationale.)

I would spend more time helping members describe what they had in mind when they suggested doing a particular activity at the next session. I am not sure that all members understood what writing a group poem would entail so they were not in a position to speak for or against the activity.

Review Questions

1. Will the leadership functions of the development stage be much the same as that of the formation stage?
2. What types of control and power issues are characteristic of this stage? Is the role of the leader to assume the responsibility to solve these issues?
3. What are some of the factors interacting in a group at a given moment? At a concrete level? At a symbolic level?
4. How may a leader encourage group members to assume various group membership roles?
5. Is testing the safety of the group still an issue for members in the development stage? If so, what group actions can be taken to meet this need? How may a leader alter the group's structure to influence the group's process? Can the activity itself be useful in influencing the group's process?

References

Bradford, L. P., Stock, D., and Horwitz, M. (1978). How to diagnose group problems. In L. P. Bradford (ed.), Group Development (2nd ed.), pp. 62–78. La Jolla, CA: University Associates.

Cartwright, D., and Zander, A. (1968). Motivational processes in groups: Introduction. In D. Cartwright and A. Zander (eds.), Group Dynamics Research and Theory (3rd ed.), pp. 401–417. New York: Harper & Row.

Cohen, A. M., and Smith, R. D. (1976). The Critical Incident in Growth Groups: Theory and Technique. La Jolla, CA: University Associates.

Corey, G., and Corey, M. S. (1982). Groups: Process and Practice (2nd ed.). Monterey, CA: Brooks/Cole.

Csikszentmihalyi, M. (1975). Beyond Boredom and Anxiety: The Experience of Play in Work and Games. San Francisco: Jossey-Bass.

Garland, J. A., and Frey, L. A. (1970). Application of stages of group development to groups in psychiatric settings. In S. Bernstein (ed.), Further Explorations in Group Work, pp. 1–28. Boston: Boston University School of Social Work.

Garland, J. A., Jones, H. E., and Kolodny, R. L. (1973). A model for stages of development in social work groups. In S. Bernstein (ed.), Explorations in Group Work: Essays in Theory and Practice, pp. 17–71. Boston: Milford House.

Henry, A. D., Nelson, D. L., and Duncombe, L. W. (1984). Choice making in group and individual activity. American Journal of Occupational Therapy 38(4): 245–251.

Klein, A. F. (1972). Effective Groupwork: An Introduction to Principle and Method. New York: Association Press.

Miles, M. B. (1981). Learning to Work in Groups: A Practical Guide for Members and Trainers (2nd ed.). New York: Teachers College Press.

Yerxa, E. J. (1967). 1966 Eleanor Clarke Slagle Lecture: Authentic occupational therapy. American Journal of Occupational Therapy 21(1): 1–9.

Chapter 9
Stage Four: Termination

Termination of a group, as in most human relationships, and especially where the participants have gone through a lot together and have developed a sense of closeness and mutuality, is fraught with sadness. It is akin to losing someone dear and feeling grief, or to feeling that one is being abandoned. It leaves one with the dread of loneliness and of having to "go it alone." It reactivates the fear of risk and the anticipation of inadequacy and hence failure. Mingled with these anxieties, if the group has been a help, are feelings of hope, of power to succeed, and of the adventure of facing a new day. (KLEIN, 1972, P. 283)

The process of termination must be viewed from two different vantage points: the termination of one member in an open group and the termination of an ongoing closed group. The issues and expectations of both cases are similar. The primary tasks of the termination stage are (1) reviewing the group experience with an accompanying consolidation of what has been learned and (2) dealing with the members' concerns and feelings about separation and loss.

The final meetings of a group are important because they give members the opportunity to clarify the meaning of their experiences in the group. This process makes members aware of what they have learned, what behaviors have changed, and what skills they may have acquired. In addition, members can decide which of these changes in behavior they can or want to bring to new situations.

In this chapter, we describe the issues a leader can expect to face in the termination stage. Leader functions and intervention strategies for facilitating closure are also discussed. The needs of group members with regard to action in the termination stage will be highlighted. Finally, the principles discussed are applied to three case studies through completed group session plans and session evaluation forms for the termination stage.

Issues and Expectations

The leader should expect certain reactions to the termination of an individual member or the group as a whole. Although we use the term *termination* to describe this stage, we discuss the reactions in terms of their transitional roles. Termination is a transition to another stage in the life of the individuals involved; therefore, the leader must guide the members into that new stage. Dealing with the following issues and reactions to termination will enable members to move beyond the group.

Denial and Avoidance

Group members may deny the reality of termination (Cohen and Smith, 1976; Klein, 1972) by not talking about it or by putting off confronting their feelings until the last few minutes when it is too late to discuss them thoroughly. Groups may also deny the reality of termination by making elaborate plans for the group to meet again in a reunion. In such a case, the end of the group sessions is acknowledged, but the end of the group relationship is denied.

Premature Termination

Typically, some members will withdraw from the group before issues of termination are discussed. Withdrawal is manifest through lack of participation (Cohen and Smith, 1976; Corey and Corey, 1982), lateness, or absenteeism.

Anxiety and Fear

It is quite common for group members to experience anxiety over the impending termination (Cohen and Smith, 1976; Corey and Corey, 1982; Klein, 1972).

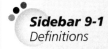

Fears usually concern the members' ability to transfer what they have learned in the group to outside situations. Such anxiety may manifest itself in regressed behavior, moving apart from the group to gain closure, or a return to behavior stereotypic of the formation and development stages of the group.

Depression and Anger

Feelings of anger may surface around the time of termination. At times, this anger is not expressed and the grief is internalized; hence, members feel depressed and abandoned (Klein, 1972). The anger may also be directed toward the group in general for not having fulfilled the fantasies or goals of the member. Similarly, the anger may be directed toward the leader or the institution. Members may view the group experience as worthless and become irritated with one another.

Sadness

As the group members seek closure, members may experience intense sadness (Cohen and Smith, 1976; Klein, 1972). As a result, members may reduce the intensity of their involvement.

Raising New Issues for Discussion

Some members, under the pressure of termination, may bring up new issues for the group to consider when there is no longer time to discuss these issues adequately. It is important for leaders to be aware of this possibility and to acknowledge the importance of the issue. In addition, they must be realistic: They must point out the inappropriateness of dealing with new agendas at the time of closure.

Leader Functions and Intervention Strategies

The most important response of the leader to member reactions is to continue to acknowledge feelings as done throughout the group meetings.

Encouraging Members to Express Concerns

As in the early phases of the group, the leader needs to encourage expression of fears and expectations as members reach the final sessions of the group.

These feelings may be as troubling to the members as were their initial feelings upon entering the group. The task of the leader is to remind the members that the cohesiveness and support they feel in the group today is the result of their participation in the group process. The leader should remind the group that each member contributed to creating the atmosphere they now experience.

Discussing Feelings of Loss, Anger, and Sadness

If the leader avoids dealing with feelings of loss and anger at the end of the group, members probably will avoid doing so also. The leader must facilitate an open discussion of the feelings of loss that accompany the end of any meaningful experience. If they are not openly discussed, members will react with feelings of anxiety, depression, and anger.

Dealing With Unfinished Business

The leader must allot time for going over and discussing unfinished business relating to transactions between members or to the group process or goals (Corey and Corey, 1982). Members may need to bring up unresolved conflicts with other members or with the leader. It is not always possible to resolve the issues that are raised, but an exploration of their current state can be helpful before the group terminates. Member needs and resources should also be assessed so that appropriate referrals can be made when necessary.

Review of Members' Participation in the Group

Members have been giving and receiving feedback throughout the life of the group, and that has helped them to assess their impact on the group. During the last sessions, more specific feedback may be helpful as part of a review of each member's participation. This process might be prefaced by asking members to report briefly how they saw themselves acting in the group and what the group has meant to them. This activity can be followed by feedback from the group concerning how they have perceived each member's participation in the group.

Transfer of Learning to New Situations

The termination stage can be a time for members to prepare for the new experiences that they will encounter in new situations or groups. The knowledge or skills they have gained from this group experience may help them cope with new situations. In the final sessions members are prepared to generalize their experiences and to relate them to situations outside the group. To integrate their experiences, Corey and Corey (1982) have suggested such activities as role playing and behavioral rehearsal.

Reinforcing Confidentiality

At the time of termination the leader should repeat the principle of confidentiality and remind members to respect confidences even after the group has ended.

Members' Action Responses

The issues raised in the termination stage lead to the membership needs related to action shown in Table 9-1. To support purposeful action, the leader should provide structure and encourage members to assume group maintenance roles. This is especially important because closure can activate withdrawal or strong emotions in people. These feelings may prompt members to return to behaviors displayed in the formation and development stages of the group. Hence, the ac-

Table 9-1
Group Membership Needs Related to Action: Termination Stage

Termination Stage Issues	Purposeful Action	Self-Initiated Action	Spontaneous (Here-and-Now) Action	Group-Centered Action	Leader Skills Employed
Denial and avoidance Premature termination	More focus on mainte-nance roles and less on task	Moving apart from group	Becoming more individual centered Less focus on here and now; more review of group's history and life	Withdrawal	Confrontation Modeling behavior Feedback
Anxiety and fear		Trust versus mistrust Power struggles		Devalue importance of group and learnings	
Depression and anger		Regressive behavior Conflicts with leader and other members		Anger toward leader Group con-flicts pre-dominate Lack of partici-pation	Genuineness and empathy Listening and responding Reality testing Self-disclosure Feedback
Sadness		Withdrawal from group Feedback to other members with less intensity		Silences and inactivity	
Raising new issues for discussion	More structure Closure	Regressive		Viewing work done as worthless	Reality testing Confrontation

tion is centered on individual member's needs rather than on the group's needs. Members' responses are less spontaneous, and group interactions focus on conflicts with the leader or with one another. Such responses require the leader to use the full range of skills described and noted in Table 9-1.

Leader Emotional Response

As in other periods of growth, the termination stage raises many feelings and reactions. Both group members and the leader may feel a sense of accomplishment coupled with anxiety as well as sadness over the loss of a group. The leader may experience feelings similar to those at the group's formation or when a member joined the group. If leaders have a positive experience with a group or an individual terminating, they will likely feel some sadness and happiness for gains made. The leader may also experience a sense of relief if the process went badly.

Sometimes, a member or group must end before being ready. This may be because a person moves, a schedule changes, or reimbursement is insufficient or time-limited. There are also situations in which a therapist must ask a group member to leave a group. The person may be unable to handle the expectations of the group for example, or an alternative modality may be more appropriate. Leaders' reactions will, of course, vary in relation to the particular group and member but also in relation to their own history and experience with loss and change. Further, people react differently to success as well as not meeting a challenge. These reactions will get stirred as the therapist helps individuals as well as a group get closure.

It is most important that the leader or coleaders be aware of their experience and monitor personal reactions so as not to interfere with the growth of members. Self-reflective questions (Box 9-1) can help leaders to self-examine their emotional responses and to identify patterns in their own reactions to

---

Box 9-1
Leader Self-Reflective Questions

- Do I feel the group or individual is ready to terminate? Is my appraisal consistent with the group member's perceptions or others significant to the person such as family members?

- If the former appraisal is inconsistent, where is my reaction coming from? Is my satisfaction, disappointment, or relief relevant and appropriate from the member's perspective?

- How much of my response is useful to share? Am I assisting the member in a helpful way to make a transition from the group to functioning without the support, or with other types of help?

- What have I learned from working with this group or individuals in the group?

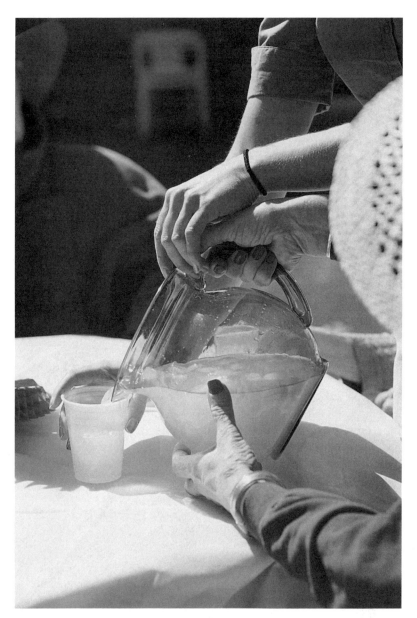

Figure 9-1. Consolidating group experience. (Photograph by Sarah Brezinsky.)

working in the termination stage (see Case Studies 1, 2, and 3 Session Evaluation Form Protocols). The degree to which the leader shares reactions will vary
according to the type of group and the theoretical model. Settings also have cultures by which to judge supportive ways to bring a group to ending. Schools,
for example, have many ceremonial structures in which people share their feel-

ings about termination such as graduation exercises. The length as well as intensity of the relationships, member's needs and the therapist's own degree of comfort are equally important measures for calibrating the degree of self-disclosure that is appropriate.

Conclusion

The termination of any role or relationship is difficult, and the leader must carefully guide the members in dealing with this stage. At this point, members must make the final effort to absorb and consolidate their experiences to move forward and continue their progress. With the help of the leader, many members view this stage as a true transition from therapy to life outside the group. In the following pages, the principles are applied in the completed group session plans and the session evaluation forms for the two case studies. See Fig. 9-1.

CASE STUDY NUMBER 1
Open Occupational Therapy Group

Separating From the Group in the Termination Stage

Group Session Plan Protocol

A. Name of Group   Project Group

Date   June 19

B. Specific goals for the group session
To enhance self-esteem.
To increase interest in avocational activities.

C. Specific goals for group members if different from those just listed and goals for each group member
Group members: Express feelings of loss, anger, and sadness.
Terminating the member: Express fears about leaving group; review work in group; and discuss concerns about returning to job/family.

D. Description of and rationale for methods and procedures
Encourage group to complete terrariums started in prior session.
Remind group that the member is leaving today.
Encourage group members to discuss their feelings and reactions to the member leaving.
Plan for following session by asking each member to share what they have learned in group and what their future goals are.
Rationale: Completing the group activity should enhance members' sense of efficacy and joy in avocational tasks. It gives members a behavioral scheme for a similar activity outside of the hospital. Members may deny or avoid intense feelings that surface around termination. Explor-

ing the issues will help members externalize their feelings, get support, and see the value of involvement in action with others. Planning for the next session gives members remaining in the group a sense of hope and continuity.

E. **Description of and rationale for leadership role**
Listen and reflect members' feelings back to group.
Check if perceptions are accurate.

Rationale: Members may conceal their feelings of anger and sadness about a member leaving the group or of feeling hopeless because of being left in the group.

Encourage members to review the group's progress by summarizing some of the recent events and asking the group to add their reflections.

Rationale: This should reinforce what has been learned in group and center the responsibility for future action and planning on the group members.

Ask members to report what the group has meant to them.
Rationale: This gives members an opportunity to transfer what they learned in the group to outside situations and deal with unfinished business with the departing member or group leaders.

F. **Description of necessary preparations**
Unlock and open doors to occupational therapy room and supply cabinet.
Review plan with coleader.

G. **List of material and equipment needed**
Small plants, potting soil, colored gravel, spoons, water, newspaper, and plastic cups

H. **Time and sequence outline for session, including what you will say and do as leader and what the group will do; consider both content and process**
Review of group plan for session and announcement of member's termination (approximately 5 minutes).
Completion of terrariums (approximately 25 minutes).
Discussion: Member termination, progress review, and planning (approximately 15 minutes).

I. **Other information pertinent to this specific session**

For example: Will there be any new members, coleaders, or guests? Is there an unusual tone on the unit or special event that is about to occur or just occurred for the individual member or group?
The member who is departing from group has attended 10 sessions.
Group members learned yesterday that the chief psychiatrist on the inpatient unit is leaving to assume a position in another hospital.
New psychiatry residents are expected to arrive on July 1, along with other student interns in psychology and social work.

An occupational therapy student is observing the group today. The members do not know her.

A. **Name of Group**   Project Group

Date   June 19

B. **Were the goals accomplished? (Give rationale and state outcome.)**
Partially. Members expressed their anger about being in the hospital and fears regarding going home. They reluctantly completed their projects and disparagingly commented on their self-worth and the value of avocations.

Was the session helpful in accomplishing short-term and long-term group and individual member goals?
Yes, in regard to long-term group goals: members recognized and supported each other's feelings. No, in regard to improved self-esteem and avocational role interest.

Do you have any evidence that the session(s) have been helpful to the members' functioning (adaptation) outside of the group?
Yes, members asked for evening passes to go to the movies.

C. **Was the group structure adequate for accomplishing the goals? Give rationale and consider: leadership; time/length of meeting; open versus closed group; time, sequence, methods, and procedures; media/modalities/techniques employed; norms/behaviors reinforced implicitly or explicitly; methods of reinforcement; and stage of group's development.**
Given the many staff changes and member termination, it would have been preferable to have a group discussion before the task component of the session.

Did the structure provide optimal "action" or "flow activity" for a "flow state" to occur?
No. Members were feeling abandoned and self-doubting. By first completing the terrarium project, members' here-and-now reactions were diverted from reality testing and getting group support.

Did the structure provide optimal purposeful, self-initiated, spontaneous, and group-centered "action" for cognitive and emotional impact, skill learning, and adaptation to occur through "occupation" (Box 9-2)?
Yes. The opportunity to discuss feelings, summarize events, and plan for

---

Box 9-2
Providing Insight

Leaders should ask what they would do differently the next time.

the future enabled the group to free themselves for other activities later in the day.

Did the structure provide for new learning, reinforcement of current level of functioning or adaptation, or did it reinforce functioning below current level of adaptation? Explain and give rationale.
The structure provided members an opportunity to learn how feelings can get in the way of action if they are used to reinforce a sense of passivity and helplessness rather than to assert oneself by communicating needs.

Did the structure provide an opportunity for evaluation and feedback regarding the group procedures and member progress? Explain.
Yes. The group discussion at the end of the session encouraged members to give each other feedback.

D. **What changes would you make regarding group goals and structure for the next session, or if you were to lead this session again?**
I would allow silence to persist and be examined before intervening by prompting the group to complete the activity task.

E. **Were you adequately prepared for the session? (Give rationale, considering such things as time, place, materials, and physical and emotional environment.)**
The physical environment was adequate; however, the emotional climate was not. The group members were on the verge of discussion rather than proceeding with the task. The session was too highly structured for the emotional content that came forth.

F. **How did you function as leader? How did your behavior and role affect the group? Were you effective? (Give rationale.) What did you learn about yourself as group leader?**
I believe that if the emotional content were dealt with first, the group would have had more of a sense of success with their products. I learned that "listening" to the group is particularly essential in the first minutes of a session and that the session should then be adapted accordingly. By not listening, I implicitly gave the message that feelings were not important.

G. **Was the group interaction as you anticipated? If problems occurred, what processes can you identify as a basis for understanding the problems?**
I did not anticipate how angry and abandoned the members felt. Two members exploded at the student observer and said she was not welcome. The many changes on the unit seem to have decreased the feeling of safety in the group and precipitated a regression to issues regarding trust versus mistrust.

H. **In the future, what might you do differently as group leader? (Give rationale.)**

I would actively listen to the members before encouraging them to complete the task. This would create more open communication and, hopefully, a match between member needs and the task.

CASE STUDY NUMBER 2
Closed Occupational Therapy Group

Revival of Formation Stage Issues in the Termination Stage

Group Session Plan Protocol

A. **Name of Group**   Energy Conservation/Time Management Group

   Date   Eighth session out of eight—December 20

B. **Specific goals for the group session**
   To establish a resource network among group members.
   To evaluate the group.
   To express feelings regarding discharge and group's termination.

C. **Specific goals for group members if different from those just listed and goals for each group member**
   To symbolize group's gains and termination by having a party.

D. **Description of and rationale for methods and procedures**
   Share home phone numbers.
   Review various community resources.
   Have members bake cookies and prepare fruit salad.
   Rationale: To reinforce gains and ability to be independent; to provide concrete resources.

E. **Description of and rationale for leadership role**
   Listen and convey empathy.
   Reality test; clarify feelings.
   Rationale: To bring closure to group in a supportive manner.

F. **Describe necessary preparations**
   Buy ingredients for cookies and salad.
   Schedule use of kitchen.

G. **List material and equipment needed**
   Flour, sugar, eggs, butter, chocolate chips, bowls, adaptive utensils, fruit, napkins, and plates

H. **Time and sequence outline for session, including what you will say and do as leader and what the group will do; consider both content and process**
   Prepare food.

Discussion (farewell and resources).

Eat food and clean up.

I. Other information pertinent to this specific session: For example: Will there be any new members, coleaders, or guests? Is there an unusual tone on the unit or special event that is about to occur or just occurred for the individual member or group?

None.

Session Evaluation Form Protocol

A. **Name of Group**   Energy Conservation/Time Management Group

   Date   December 20

B. **Were the goals accomplished? (Give rationale and state outcome.)**

   Yes. Members prepared food for party. Expressed their sadness and joys of accomplishments in group; thoughts about returning to community and resources they might use.

   Was the session helpful in accomplishing short-term and long-term group and individual member goals?

   Yes, for the most part. However, two members were somewhat silent and withdrawn from group.

   Do you have any evidence that the session(s) have been helpful to the members' functioning (adaptation) outside of the group?

   Yes. Families have reported interest in meeting other members of group when patient returns home.

C. **Was the group structure adequate for accomplishing the goals? Give rationale and consider: leadership; time/length of meeting; open versus closed group; time, sequence, methods, and procedures; media/modalities/techniques employed; norms/behaviors reinforced implicitly or explicitly; methods of reinforcement; and stage of group's development.**

   Yes, except for two withdrawn members. These members needed more active encouragement to share their feelings.

   Did the structure provide optimal "action" or "flow activity" for a "flow state" to occur? (Box 9-3).

   Yes. Members laughed and cried spontaneously. They also tolerated moments of silence together.

Box 9-3
Allowing Flow

The group structure must provide optimal "action" or "flow activity" for a "flow state" to occur.

Did the structure provide optimal purposeful, self-initiated, spontaneous, and group-centered "action" for cognitive and emotional impact, skill learning, and adaptation to occur through "occupation"?

Yes. The cooking/baking allowed members to successfully practice what they learned and in a culturally appropriate way share their feelings about the group's termination.

Did the structure provide for new learning, reinforcement of current level of functioning or adaptation, or did it reinforce functioning below current level of adaptation? Explain and give rationale.

For the most part, members learned that they can get more support by sharing and initiating action. They were required to complete an activity using newly acquired task and social-emotional skills.

Did the structure provide an opportunity for evaluation and feedback regarding the group procedures and member progress? Explain.

Yes. The session was planned to focus on termination and evaluation, so members were prepared to evaluate.

D. **What changes would you make regarding group goals and structure for the next session, or if you were to lead this session again?**

I would have a written evaluation form so that the less verbal members would have an easier time giving feedback.

E. **Were you adequately prepared for the session? (Give rationale, considering such things as time, place, materials, and physical and emotional environment.)**

For the most part, yes (see comment under "D").

F. **How did you function as leader? How did your behavior and role affect the group? Were you effective? (Give rationale.) What did you learn about yourself as group leader?**

By my being supportive, task-oriented, and empathetic, members were able to accomplish a task, and most shared their concerns and sorrow.

G. **Was the group interaction as you anticipated? If problems occurred, what processes can you identify as a basis for understanding the problems?**

I did not anticipate the withdrawal of two members. The discussion of closure appeared to revive feelings of distrust and anxiety present in these two members in the first few group sessions.

H. **In the future, what might you do differently as group leader? (Give rationale.)**

I would take a more active role in involving the silent members and discuss the goals of each session earlier in the group. Perhaps a posted schedule of the group's goals, unit activities, and session goals would be useful to members.

CASE STUDY NUMBER 3
Community-Based Occupational Therapy Group

Reactions to Termination—Denial, Fear, and Withdrawal

GROUP SESSION PLAN PROTOCOL

A. Name of Group   Activity Group

Date   September 27, last session of 10.

B. Specific goals for the group session
To address group and individual member feelings regarding termination.
To evaluate the group experience.
To increase initiative and interest in avocational activities.
To increase socialization between members.

C. Specific goals for group members if different from those mentioned already and goals for each group member
None.

D. Description of and rationale for methods and procedures
Remind members that this is their last group meeting.
Help them to engage in a group-centered activity that will recapture their sense of closeness and allow them to discuss their feelings and concerns.
A collage of memorable events in the group's history will provide a way to recap their experiences and stages of growth of the group.
Members will have to use their own initiative to decide which events will be portrayed in the collage.

E. Description of and rationale for leadership role
Encourage members to review the group's progress and concretize these events in the collage (both serious and humorous).
Rationale: To reinforce what has been learned and enjoyed in the group
Listen and reflect members' feelings back to the group and ask for feedback on their accuracy.
Rationale: Members may conceal their feelings about separation from the group.

F. Describe necessary preparations
Discuss and formulate plans for session with aide. Role of aide will be to assist, as needed, with the collage (task). The role of the leader will be to deal primarily with the concerns and feelings of members.
Materials for the collage will be available on the table.

G. List material and equipment needed
Large construction paper for collage, magazines, precut magazine pictures, stickers, colored pencils, glue, and scissors

H. Time and sequence outline for sessions, including what you will do and say as leader and what the group will do; consider both content and process

1. Greetings and distribution of name tags; review of the group plan for the session and reminder that this is the last session of the group (approximately 10 minutes).
2. Review of last meeting and group discussion and corrections (approximately 5 minutes).
3. Introduction of the activity, a collage representing memories of the group sessions. The group is to choose the exact theme for the collage and the process for completing it. The group has already made a collage, so members are familiar with the process, but the leader will briefly describe the process again. Leader suggests that they might want to work in pairs to construct the collage sections (approximately 20 minutes).
4. Planning of the collage; members work in pairs to find selected materials and to complete the collage (approximately 20 minutes).
5. Viewing the finished collage and discussion among members about what they wished to represent in their section of the collage (approximately 10 minutes).
6. Processing of the session and a review of the learning that members have experienced in the group. Leader also allows time for the expression of feelings regarding the termination of the group (approximately 30 minutes).

I. Other information pertinent to this specific session: For example: Will there be any new members, coleaders, or guests? Is there an unusual tone on the unit or special event that is about to occur or just occurred for the individual member or group?
None.

Session Evaluation Form Protocol

A. Name of Group   Activity Group

Date   October 2, 10:00 AM to 11:30 AM. Tenth and final session of a closed group.

B. Were the goals accomplished? (Give rationale and state outcome.)
Yes, all the goals were accomplished.
1. The activity stimulated conversation and socialization between group members and increased their initiative and interest in avocational activities.
2. The final section of the session, when members discussed the activity and reflected on their learning during the ten weeks, helped them to address the group experience and their feelings about termination.

Was the session helpful in accomplishing short-term and long-term group and individual member goals?

Partially. Some of the members remained quiet and withdrawn from the group, much less involved than other members.

Do you have any evidence that the session(s) have been helpful to the members' functioning (adaptation) outside of the group?
Yes. Families have reported increased involvement and initiative in family matters. Some group members are now having lunch together after the morning group.

C. **Was the group structure adequate for accomplishing the goals? Give rationale, and consider: leadership; time/length of meeting; open versus closed group; time, sequence, methods and procedures; media/modalities/techniques employed; norms/behaviors reinforced implicitly or explicitly; methods of reinforcement; and stage of group's development.**
Yes. The closed group, length, procedures and methods of reinforcement were adequate. The modalities employed were perhaps too difficult, in places, for the more frail and withdrawn members of the group, who were more at a stage of parallel than cooperative development.

Did the structure provide optimal "action" or "flow activity" for a "flow state" to occur?
See "D" below.

Did the structure provide optimal purposeful, self-initiated, spontaneous, and group-centered "action" for cognitive and emotional impact, skill learning, and adaptation to occur through "occupation"?
Yes, the reminiscing and collage allowed group members to be actively involved in sharing experiences and then in a group-centered activity such as making a collage.

Did the structure provide for new learning or reinforcement of current level of functioning or adaptation, or did it reinforce functioning below current level of adaptation? Explain and give rationale.
Most of the members learned to take more initiative in the activity sessions, and that they could help each other to work successfully as a group. The structure supported the overall goal, reinforcement of current maximum level of individual functioning.

Did the structure provide an opportunity for evaluation and feedback regarding the group procedures and member progress? Explain.
Yes. There was always enough time at the end of the session for feedback and evaluation of group and member progress. The session included a discussion of the level of enjoyment and satisfaction of members. This session was planned to focus on termination so members were prepared to talk about their feelings about the group's end.

D. **What changes would you make regarding group goals and structure for the next session, or if you were to lead this session again?**
Given the opportunity to repeat history, I would not change group goals or structure. As happens in many community-based groups where there

is little opportunity for screening of participants, the level of group performance may be varied; therefore, group activities may be too advanced, or too elementary, for all group members. This did occur in one session of this group when one woman commented that she was tired of "cutting and pasting like in kindergarten." Members could participate in the activity today at a number of different levels, both on the task and the emotional level.

E. Were you adequately prepared for the session? (Give rationale, considering such things as time, place, materials, and physical and emotional environment.)

Yes. We were prepared to make changes in the activity in response to member comments or emotional reactions.

F. How did you function as leader? How did your behavior and role affect the group? Were you effective? (Give rationale.) What did you learn about yourself as group leader?

My leadership style was democratic and supportive. This style seemed to enable members to complete the task and share their feelings about termination.

G. Was the group interaction as you anticipated? If problems occurred, what processes can you identify as a basis for understanding the problems?

When I sensed the withdrawal of Tom and the increased agitation on the part of Agnes, I reassured members of the group that it was safe for them to express their feelings and I modeled this by expressing some of my own feelings.

H. In the future, what might you do differently as group leader? (Give rationale.)

I felt that this was a successful group. Some of the members would benefit from a longer group experience. I would redesign the group without setting a firm time limit. I would have a graduation day after ten sessions for those members who are ready to join other groups and let the others continue in this group for another 10 weeks.

Review Questions

1. How may issues of termination differ for an open group versus a closed group?
2. What is the primary task of the termination stage?
3. What are some of the ways that group members deal with the termination experience?
4. What is the role of the leader in helping members deal with their feelings? What happens if there is no discussion of these feelings?
5. What are the activity goals for the termination stage? How can these activities help the members to review their participation and experiences in the group?

6. Is the group action of the termination stage centered primarily on group needs or on individual member needs? What leader skills are useful in this process?

References

Cohen, A. M., and Smith, R. D. (1976). The Critical Incident in Growth Groups: Theory and Technique. La Jolla, CA: University Associates.

Corey, G., and Corey, M. S. (1982). Groups: Process and Practice (2nd ed.). Monterey, CA: Brooks/Cole.

Klein, A. F. (1972). Effective Groupwork: An Introduction to Principle and Method. New York: Association Press.

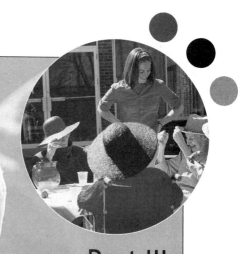

Part III
Teaching and Research

In the first section of this book, we present descriptive historical and research data on groups in general and on occupational therapy groups in particular. We then outline our model for group treatment called the functional group model. The second section of this book is devoted to the application of the functional model to therapy groups and addresses in particular the role of the group leader. In this third section, we consider the professional areas that our model for practice relies on for acknowledgment and validation: education and research.

The functional group is the first model for group treatment to be developed in the field of occupational therapy (Box 10-1). Continuing research and evaluation will undoubtedly bring forth new evidence on the effectiveness of various techniques, and this evidence, in turn, will lead to modification of the concepts and principles that guide group work. The practice of group work in occupational therapy will continue to be defined and recognized through the education of therapists and the collection of research data. Anyone who develops competence in a particular field recognizes that competence must be polished, advanced, and improved. To master a particular model and its application is only the beginning of a longer journey toward its full use in helping individuals achieve their goals and meet their needs. As part of this process, the therapist will undoubtedly look to the research literature and to educational resources.

Chapter **10**
Concluding Remarks:
Teaching and Research

Functional Group Model

This chapter begins with a discussion on clinical reasoning. This is appropriate because the functional group is a conceptual model rather than a frame of reference. Its application is inductive and informs practice. It does not dictate *a priori* what that practice should be. Likewise, the model originated from our experiences leading groups and teaching courses on group process and was not an outgrowth of one theory or frame of reference in occupational therapy.

Three types of reasoning have been found to guide occupational therapy practice: procedural, interactive, and conditional modes (Fleming, 1991). According to Fleming (1991):

> The procedural reasoning strategy was used when the therapist thought about the person's physical ailments and what procedures were appropriate to alleviate them. Interactive reasoning was used to help the therapist interact with and understand the person better. Conditional reasoning, a complex form of social reasoning, was used to help the patient in the difficult process of reconstructing a life now permanently changed by injury or disease. (p. 1007)

Box 10-1
Research-Based

The model is based on the evidence of current research in the field of group treatment and group dynamics, and in occupational therapy.

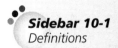

Sidebar 10-1
Definitions

Procedural reasoning: *Therapeutic strategy that addresses the patient's physical ailments and procedures that can alleviate them*

Interactive reasoning: *Therapeutic strategy that helps the therapist interact with and understand the patient better*

Conditional reasoning: *Therapeutic strategy that helps the patient reconstruct a life permanently changed by injury or disease*

Discussions and data-based research on the functional group model augment understanding for the interactive and conditional reasoning of occupational therapists. Fleming (1991) explains that "in using conditional reasoning, the therapist appears to reflect on the success or failure of the clinical encounter from both the procedural and interactive standpoints and attempts to integrate the two" (p. 1012). Several examples of how a therapist might "imagine how the condition could change" (Fleming, 1991, p. 1012) are gleaned from the model. For example, Persson (1996) observes how the demands of occupational activities in an activity group can influence participants' experience of "play and flow." Haiman (1990) suggests using the General Plan Protocol as a step in decision making about group structure and content. Similarly, Borg and Bruce (1991) mention that planning an activity in the functional group model is a cognitive strategy for leader intervention. In a university setting, Scott (1999) uses the group protocol session plan and Session Evaluation Form Protocol as tools for developing group leadership skills in occupational therapy students. Falk-Kessler, Momich, and Perel (1991) support our notion of therapeutic factors as important to planning effective occupational therapy groups. Although based in the Model of Human Occupation and viewed as appropriate for individuals more minimally functioning, Kaplan's "Directive Group" is purported as similar in aim to the functional group in regard to assisting adaptation through purposeful, self-initiated, spontaneous, and group-centered action (Kaplan, 1988). Further support that functional group concepts be considered in conditional reasoning comes from Posthuma (1989). She emphasizes the importance of group size, number of staff and influence on interaction, and relevance of our suggested use of the sociogram and Bales Interaction Process Analysis. Kielhofner (1992, 1997) fully incorporates the model in his articulation of conceptual models in occupational therapy. He gives emphasis to conditional and interactive aspects in carefully outlining our arguments of "therapeutic intervention" and "technology for application." Bruce (1988) gives more attention to interactive reasoning aspects in her recognition of the model's intent of focusing on such things as here-and-now aspects of interaction and an individual's strengths.

The widely acclaimed University of Southern California Well Elderly Research Study (Clark and colleagues, 1997; Jackson and colleagues, 1998; Mandel and colleagues, 1999) provides strong support for the effectiveness of group programs using the functional group model in preparation of occupational therapist leaders. In this large-scale randomized effectiveness study, an occupation-based group program was found to be highly successful in influencing the physical and mental health, occupational functioning, and life satisfaction of a culturally diverse population of well elders. Both the philosophical base in occupational science and the therapeutic process used in the lifestyle redesign modular group program are thoroughly consistent with tenets of the functional group model. The well elderly study program model is a design well suited for replication with other populations.

Interestingly, researchers (Glass, Mendes de Leon, Marottoli, and Berkman, 1999) in a recent large-scale, population-based, 13-year study of elderly, confirmed the importance of social engagement and productive activity in relation to successful aging. They found social activity was as responsible for lowering the risk of mortality as were fitness activities. They speculated that activity may confer survival benefits through psychosocial pathways more than thought earlier. The authors suggested that public policy measures support programs that reduce barriers to social engagement. They also mentioned a study by Teasdale, Christensen, and Pinner (1993) in which occupational therapy intervention showed the feasibility of increasing levels of leisure and social activity in cranial trauma and stroke patients. One hopes to see a proliferation of occupational therapy groups as the link between survival and social activity is further documented (Box 10-2).

Two additional outcomes of the functional group model are worthy of mention. First, our historical analysis of group work in occupational therapy has been used as part of descriptions of the profession's history and for justifying group treatment as a legitimate modality in occupational therapy (Falk-Kessler, Momich, and Perel, 1991; Haiman, 1990; Nelson et al., 1988; Posthuma, 1989; Stein and Tallant, 1988; Tallant, 1998). Second, the survey

---

Box 10-2
Lasting Legacy

The functional group model has been used to:

- Help describe the official history of occupational therapy
- Justifiy group treatment as part of occupational therapy
- Analyze trends in practice
- Identify research areas
- Support group work practice in occupational therapy

of practice and model (Duncombe and Howe, 1985; Howe and Schwartzberg, 1986) has been employed to analyze trends in practice, identify research areas, and support group work practice in the profession (Barnes and Schwartzberg, in press; Barnes and Schwartzberg, 1999; Borg and Bruce, 1991; Brinson and Kannenberg, 1996; Brown, 1990; Bruce and Borg, 1993; Bruce, 1988; Cara and MacRae, 1998; Cole, 1998; Cottrell, 1993; Duncombe and Howe, 1995; Eklund, 1996; Kaplan, 1986; Kielhofner, 1992; McDermott, 1988; Persson, 1996; Posthuma, 1989, 1996; Schwartzberg, 1993, 1998, 1999; Schwartzberg and Abeles, 1986; Scott, 1999; Steffan and Nelson, 1987).

Research on group treatment and group work in occupational therapy has expanded since the first edition of this book was published in 1986. Some studies directly sought to verify aspects of the functional group model, whereas others more indirectly explain related phenomena. In the next section, research implications and some studies pertinent to the functional group model are reviewed.

Research

There are relatively few research studies on group treatment and group work in occupational therapy, although the number has certainly grown over the past two decades. This should not be surprising, because the field is young and there are still many problems in conducting research with groups (Box 10-3). In outcome studies, for instance, the standard controls for error are practically impossible to impose, because each group may be expected to respond differently because of its unique developmental context. The fact that no two groups are alike poses problems of replication. Furthermore, ethical and professional considerations complicate research design and restrict research opportunities. Despite these problems, important research studies in occupational therapy group work were published, and several of these deserve special consideration. From these studies, inferences concerning the functional group can be drawn.

Researchers have been primarily concerned with the relationship between factors of group process and the group format. The research findings can be organized around two questions relevant to verification of the functional group model:

- What influence does group format have on the quality and quantity of interaction, meaning assigned to the group action, and members' functional status?

Box 10-3
Defying Categorization

A group is, by definition, a dynamic entity that involves a number of interpersonal variables that defy the usual controls applied to research studies.

- What influence does the group format have on the cost-effectiveness of the treatment?

Group Format

Schwartzberg, Howe, and McDermott (1982) undertook a descriptive study of three treatment group formats in an acute inpatient psychiatric unit of a general hospital. The researchers sought to identify and analyze patterns in the quality and quantity of verbal interaction in these groups. The groups studied were a community group meeting, a self-expression group that was a combination of task-oriented and process-oriented occupational therapy group treatment, and an open occupational therapy group in which patients could choose and carry out individual activities. Results showed that the open occupational therapy group had a significantly greater amount of person-to-person communication than did the other two group formats and that this group also had a smaller number of patients who neither spoke nor were addressed. We may infer from this study that differences in quality and quantity of interaction are related to differences in group format (Box 10-4).

Eklund's (1999) study of treatment outcomes supports the importance of the group treatment format. She compared psychiatric outpatients receiving group-based occupational therapy with a matched group of patients receiving treatment as usual of verbal therapy. Her results indicated that the occupational therapy group was helpful for some psychiatric patients on a variety of outcome variables relating to occupational performance, global mental health, and psychiatric symptoms. The factor she isolated that separated this and other effective occupational therapy programs was a well-articulated frame of reference. In this case, Eklund inferred that the program's effectiveness resulted from conscious use of object relations theory that consistently framed the staff's behavior and therapeutic attitude.

Persson's (1996) study of play and flow furthers our understanding of the "doing" and occupational process of activity groups and directly supports the theoretical assumptions of the functional group model. In his exploratory

Box 10-4
Group Formats Studied

A study of treatment group formats in an acute inpatient psychiatric unit included:

- A community group meeting
- A self-expression group
- An open OT group

study, play and flow theory was chosen as a basis for the study of the "attention-focus" for the identification of "play/flow" [p/f] and "non-play/non-flow [np/nf] episodes" in an activity group using creative occupations with chronic pain patients. The group participants in each of the sessions were given an activity proposal structured with a different theme. All of the sessions were organized to have an introductory phase, an activity phase, and a reflection/discussion phase. Of particular significance were his findings regarding the relationship between task structure and participant states of arousal, curiosity, and attention. For example, Persson notes, "another finding from the sessions was that the frustrations of the np/nf states almost exclusively seemed to be due to the challenge presented in the tasks occasionally being experienced as too great in relation to the skills of the participants" (p. 39). Furthermore, "periods of the 'in-between state' of the participants, in this study called neutral, were more difficult to demarcate from np/nf states. . . . Between these episodes there was a gradual transition which was difficult to appraise, while the transition from the neutral to p/f episodes shows a sharper qualitative change in behaviour" (p. 39).

Kremer, Nelson, and Duncombe (1984) studied chronic psychiatric patients engaged in three different group activities in a community day treatment program. Patients were randomly assigned to three occupational therapy groups: cooking group, craft activity group, and sensory awareness activity group. After the group activity, each patient rated the affective meaning of the activity using Osgood's semantic differential scale. Results showed some differences in the affective meaning of these three activities. This research study constitutes a beginning in the long process of documenting the meaning that a particular patient population assigns to the group action.

Henry, Nelson, and Duncombe (1984) examined the affective responses of subjects to having or not having freedom of choice in engaging in a particular activity. In addition, the researchers compared the responses of subjects to completing the activity in an individual and a group setting. The subjects in this study were college students. The results indicated that there was a significant relation between choice and affective meaning for activities in the group setting. Subjects in the group with no choice of activity rated themselves as feeling significantly less powerful than those in the group who had a choice. This finding supports one of the basic assumptions of the functional group; specifically, members should be included in selecting and adapting the activity of the group.

In her discussion of the nonoccupational therapy literature on small adult task groups, Steffan (1990) identified several aspects of group format with theoretical implications for the functional group model. These variables include the following:

- Type of task, results in varying interaction profiles that affect a group's task performance (Sorenson, 1971)
- Selection of members with similar abilities, which results in better performance in cooperative group tasks (Tziner and Eden, 1985)

- Varying leadership styles, which is required in managing group conflict (Wall and Nolan, 1986)

Lundgren and Persechino (1986), using Mosey's developmental group structure for cognitive group activities in controlled social environment, found trends in improvement in memory and social interaction skills in head-injured adults.

Van Deusen and Harlowe (1987) found that in a dance program for adults with rheumatoid arthritis, a group instruction format showed significantly greater upper extremity range of motion four months after treatment. Postprogram reports found enjoyment in range of motion was significantly higher for the experimental group (ROM Dance Program) although reported frequency of exercise and rest was greater in the control group (traditional exercise and rest regimens).

Nelson and colleagues (1988) found task group structure may have a significant effect on social interaction. Groups structured in project format elicited more verbal and nonverbal interaction (members looked at each other) than groups structured in parallel fashion. Subjects were senior citizens. They cite the model regarding how determining group structure in advance (amount of sharing and creativity required) may foster or inhibit different types of social interaction or affect depending on the needs of members. This research verifies that a major role of the occupational therapy group leader is to adapt group structure to help members establish their goals. It clearly documents the "importance of task group structure." As the researchers note, "With healthy seniors as its sample, this study has demonstrated that task group structure can have a significant effect on verbal interaction, nonverbal interaction, and the perception of action in the group" (p. 28) (Box 10-5).

Steffan and Nelson (1987) found that in graduate students (female) a moderate limitation in the level of supply of the essential tools used in a stenciling activity increased group engagement. They also found it decreased conflict, but no difference in affective meaning occurred for the participants.

Froehlich and Nelson (1986) in their study did not answer whether life review in elderly individuals is better enhanced through activity or discussion. They did document the effect when a collage task was introduced in an activity group and the leader assumed the role of nondirective helper. They con-

---

Box 10-5
Efficacy of Functional Group Format

Numerous research projects demonstrated the influence of the functional group format on the quality and quantity of interaction, meaning of group action, and members' functional status.

cluded that this possibly caused each group to develop its own character and atmosphere. The activity group interacted in a positive way (talking when finished with activity) and the other in a less positive way (silence when finished and waiting).

Klyczek and Mann (1986), in a psychiatric day treatment program, found that clients receiving activity therapy versus verbal therapy achieved four times greater symptom reduction (increase in independent functioning in the community in areas of self-esteem, decision making, and others). They also noted little overall difference in community tenure between the two groups. Patients with activity therapy were hospitalized significantly more often than those with verbal therapy but for a shorter duration than the verbal therapy group.

In another study in psychiatric day treatment, DeCarlo and Mann (1985) compared the effectiveness of a verbal versus an activity group in relation to improvement in self-perceptions of interpersonal communication skills. They found "a significantly higher level of [perceived] interpersonal communication skills was attained by the activity group" (p. 20).

Cole and Greene (1988), building on studies by Schwartzberg, Howe, and McDermott (1982); Kremer, Nelson, and Duncombe (1984); and Henry, Nelson, and Duncombe (1984), compared patients (psychotic and borderline) treated in comparatively unstructured psychotherapy groups and more structured task-focused occupational therapy groups. They rejected the hypothesis that psychotic patients would respond more favorably in structured occupational therapy groups, whereas borderline patients would prefer psychotherapy groups. Data revealed preference for occupational therapy groups by both patient groups. There was considerable support for the hypothesis that psychotic patients compared with borderline patients would show less differentiated reactions across the two kinds of groups.

Greene and Cole (1991) later assessed psychiatric inpatients in terms of psychopathology level and form. Patients participated in two treatment groups. One was a psychotherapy group that was comparatively unstructured. The other group was a task-oriented group conducted by occupational therapy students. Patients were explicitly delegated what to do in developing a shared project such as planning a meal. They were directed to create different work roles to do the project. They found that the members with psychosis "tended to hold more positive views of self than borderline patients in the task groups," whereas in the psychotherapy groups those with borderline personality disorder "had higher self-regard. Also, as anticipated, the borderline patients showed greater differential reactivity to the two kinds of treatment groups" (p. 514).

Adelstein and Nelson (1985) compared effects of sharing and not sharing on affective meanings of a group collage activity in a study of university students. They found no significant differences on three factors: evaluation, power, and action.

Banning and Nelson (1987) studied the use of humor and the effect of group structure in a parallel versus project structure with female subjects. The researchers concluded that "this study has also shown that an activity structured for humor can bring people together and can influence the social climate of a small group. Group cohesion was stimulated not only in the project group involving humor but also in the parallel group involving humor" (p. 513). Banning and Nelson (1987) also noted that "another finding was that group structure (project vs. parallel) interacted with humor in a significant way. . . . The fact that activity group structure made a difference qualifies the findings of Adelstein and Nelson (1985), a study that did not find significant differences between shared-product groups (project groups) and non-shared-product groups (parallel groups)" (p. 513).

Schwartzberg (1994) sought to discern "helping factors" perceived by members in an occupational therapist facilitated, peer-developed support group. The community-based support group was found to have many of the positive attributes ascribed to processes found in successful peer support groups. These attributes included believing and feeling a part of the group, because members had the head injury as a problem in common and were able to validate the effects of the injury by sharing and receiving information through the group in a variety of ways. Legitimization, the acceptance of the head injury itself as real, appeared to be the primary factor that distinguished this group from professionally led groups. Schulz (1994) in a follow-up study, found results supporting Schwartzberg's earlier finding with some exceptions. One such difference was the concerns of the members in the first study seemed to be more problem-focused and the latter to have a broader scope. The researcher believed these differences may have resulted from the divergent research methodologies. Differences in the perspectives of the participant observer in the first study and survivors in the second may account for variations in the group studied. As occupational therapists enlarge their role in the community it would be worthwhile to continue to examine differences between the group processes and outcomes of professionally led groups versus professionally facilitated groups.

There are also several reports of the effectiveness of group treatment in the weekly occupational therapy literature. These stories include the use of occupational therapy group treatment in preparation of the geriatric client for community living (Morris, Andreassi, and Lichtenberg, 1994), stroke recovery (Marmer, 1995), hand therapy (Amini, 1999), a school-based support group for students with spinal cord injury (Rabinovitch, 1999), a role-play group for children and adolescents requiring inpatient crisis intervention (Knis, 1995), and a family support group for family members of patients hospitalized for mental illness (Locascio, 1995). Other literature of interest includes application of electronic music as an occupational therapy modality in spinal cord injury rehabilitation (Lee and Nantais, 1996), the development of a rapid rating of task group function of psychiatric patients (Margolis, Harrison, Robinson, and Jayaram, 1996), and a report of a study finding a correlation between social skills and cognitive disability that strongly suggests therapists adjust their instructional techniques in groups to both cognitive and social skill components (Stahl, 1995).

The former review, although not conclusive, does demonstrate that group format has an effect on the quality and quantity of interaction, meaning assigned to the group action, and members' functional status. It gives empirical support to beliefs held by the profession (Ross, 1987). The next question relates to the cost-effectiveness of group treatment versus individual formats in occupational therapy. This topic in the present climate of health care delivery deserves serious attention if the most people are to be served in as effective a manner possible.

Cost-Effectiveness

Using the philosophy and assumptions of the functional group, Trahey (1991) designed a "Hip Group" for patients with total hip replacements. She found that group treatment could be a cost-effective method of occupational therapy. Direct labor costs were reduced by more than one-third for patients treated primarily in group method of occupational therapy with individual treatment as an adjunct, versus traditional individual occupational therapy as primary intervention with group treatment as adjunct.

Gauthier, Dalziel, and Gauthier (1987) found group occupational therapy helped patients with Parkinson's disease maintain functional status after one year. Patients also perceived improvement in psychological well-being and had a significant decrease in bradykinesia. They concluded that group occupational therapy is valuable for patients with chronic degenerative diseases who are easily drawn into social isolation and depression. The group facilitates interaction and is more cost-effective because fewer therapists are needed.

These two studies deserve serious attention. The group format shows clear signs of being both therapeutic and cost-effective. Other studies of a similar nature may prove to be equally promising. In addition, studies of patient's perceptions of occupational therapy group treatment (Falk-Kessler, Momich, and Perel, 1991; Polimeni-Walker, Wilson, and Jewers, 1992; Webster, 1988; Webster and Schwartzberg, 1992) must also be taken into account. A recent study conducted in Sweden by Eklund (1997) showed, in addition to factors previously recognized in group psychotherapy, factors such as being occupied, being engaged in certain activities, and developing new skills are of particular therapeutic value for discharged psychiatric patients. These findings are consistent with the earlier mentioned studies and support assumptions of the functional group model. As therapists assume more community-based roles, both the outcomes and the cost-effectiveness of groups that are professionally led versus peer-led or professionally facilitated, should be examined and fees calibrated.

New and creative ways need to be developed to evaluate the outcome of different types of group treatment. Descriptive and phenomenological research designs may prove to be better suited for evaluating the complex variables found in outcome studies. Because of the increasing concern with accountability in the health care professions, research on the outcome of various approaches to treatment has become especially important. Research can also help us describe more accurately the processes within groups: cohesion, feedback, support, structure, and so on. We need greater clarification of these concepts so that they can be better understood by both practitioners and researchers. The information generated through research is crucial if therapists are to transcend the limitations of one particular model and make discerning choices among treatment alternatives.

Education

It is fitting that we should end this book with a section on education because we have been working in the field of occupational therapy education for many years. In part, the lack of educational material in the field motivated us to undertake this book. More than 40 years ago, in the proceedings of the Allenberry Conference, West (1959) reported on how group process was being taught in the occupational therapy curriculum of the time. According to a survey, the most common method used to teach group process was lecture and discussion. No research has studied how this has changed over the years.

The education for group work in occupational therapy should be oriented to the occupational context of the field. The group process and group tasks are closely related to concepts of human occupation and adaptation. An understanding of activity evaluation and analysis is indispensable to leaders and will enable them to guide the group to achieve specific treatment goals. However, an intellectual understanding of the functional group is not enough. It is essential that lecture or discussion be combined with a laboratory experience through which the student can internalize what has been learned intellectually. Only through direct experience can the student realize the power of a group and see how this power can be used to promote healing or cause trauma and pain. Through personal experience, the student develops an awareness of the importance of group acceptance, the difficulty of revealing feelings, especially positive feelings, and the courage necessary to test reality and change specific ways of behaving. Participating in a group activity as a group member provides a different experience from participation in a discussion about the activity. Finally, to view the role of the leader from the vantage point of a member provides future leaders with an understanding of the unrealistic expectations that members often have of their group leader.

Educators must also pay attention to changes in service delivery systems when preparing occupational therapists for leadership roles (Box 10-6). Community-based settings, unlike hospital-based care, may require the leader to work without a referral or control over group membership. Reimbursement for time-limited services requires that the leader be able to provide a service suitable to the type and intensity of care required by a plan of care. Further, in community settings such as schools the therapist may play more of a consultant role. However acceptable, the reimbursable format may not be in the best interests of the group member or the best of care. Given the dynamic nature of groups, this puts leaders in the very difficult position of having to document

Box 10-6
The Leader's Dilemma

Maria Domingo finds she is unable to complete progress notes for individuals in her group in the time allotted for one-to-one treatment. Without proper documentation, the service will be unreimbursed and the group program dropped. Although the group is highly cost-effective, the program is at risk unless individual outcomes are assessed and documented for third-party payment. She uses her leadership skills to influence the management team to reduce the number of initial evaluations required of therapists leading groups to allow them adequate time for documentation.

achievable goals while using a process-oriented modality. For these reasons, more than ever, the leader must learn ways to enlist members to advocate for their own care. The leader needs to be adept at moving the group from a leader-centered stance to a group-centered process.

The increased interest in more time-efficient models of treatment in managed care emphasizes the need for clarity about the mechanisms underlying the efficacy of time-limited groups (Spitz, 1999). The six elements identified as essential to brief group therapy are equally applicable to group work in occupational therapy and deserve specialized attention in curriculum. These therapeutic mechanisms are summarized in (Box 10-7). Spitz (1999) also emphasized increased patient responsibility for change and commitment to apply what is learned in the group to outside real life situations as two other critical elements for successful time-limited groups.

Box 10-7
Essential Elements

The following elements are essential to brief group therapy:

- Circumscribed focus
- Active group leadership
- Group cohesion
- Fixed-group time limits
- Contemporary present-day focus
- Careful patient selection

From: Spitz, H. (Summer 1999). Brief group psychotherapy and managed care: Integration or disconnection? The Group Solution. Newsletter of the National Registry of Certified Group Psychotherapists.

The changes described may call for the occupational therapist to have increased contact with groups such as family members and partners, community boards, and consumer groups. Information about public policy is essential to students' education as they learn to frame their practice in managed care and community-based settings. Like seasoned therapists, students will be pressed to create new arenas for practice and resist pressures to provide services at odds with the profession's code of ethics and standards of care. Beyond the occupational therapy standards of care are additional ethical concerns specifically related to group work (Box 10-8) and ethics in the managed care environment (Box 10-9). Through participation in an experiential process group, students can learn how to regulate boundaries, gain influence, and assert themselves (Box 10-10).

Box 10-8
Professional Ethics

The following are ethical considerations the professional must follow in group therapy:

- "Patients have the right to receive information about the nature of the group treatment and the possible risks."
- "The patient should be maintained in therapy only as long as clinically indicated."
- "Discrimination on the basis of race, color, gender, sexual orientation, age, religion, national origin, or physical handicap is addressed in most professional ethical guidelines and is strictly prohibited."
- "The therapist is covered by the usual guidelines regarding confidentiality, but these do not apply in the same way to the group members. The expectation of confidentiality should be spelled out in writing and repeated verbally both to the individual and to the group in the course of the first session so that it is clearly understood and the reasons appreciated."
- "Sensitive situations can arise regarding information the therapist receives from or about an individual member in the group. . . . The patient should be encouraged to bring the matter before the group himself."
- "The clinician must be aware when the needs of the patient are beyond his or her clinical competence to effectively manage. Consultation must be sought at such times and appropriate referrals made."
- "Sexual intimacy is prohibited between professional and patient."

From: MacKenzie, K. R. (Spring 1999). Professional ethics and the group psychotherapist. The Group Solution. Newsletter of the National Registry of Certified Group Psychotherapists.

Box 10-9
The Role of Clinician

The role of the clinician in managed care is carefully detailed in ethics guidelines such as the following:

- "The role of the clinician as a patient advocate should not be altered by the system of health care in which the clinician practices. This does not mean that the patient necessarily should have access to every possible treatment option, but that clinicians not be prohibited from presenting their assessment of the treatment options most indicated."

- "Healthcare system allocation guidelines that restrict choices beyond normal cost-benefit judgments should be established at a policy-making level. The clinician can then be clear about the nature of rationing guidelines and can explain these to the patient."

- "The input of clinicians should be incorporated into the process of developing service guidelines."

- "A formal, timely and accessible appeals mechanism should be in place for situations in which the clinician believes a serious clinical error is possible."

- "The focus should be on cost-effective delivery of health care, not on arbitrary withholding of care."

- "Patients should be fully informed about benefit limitations."

From: MacKenzie, K. R. (Spring 1999). Professional ethics and the group psychotherapist. The Group Solution. Newsletter of the National Registry of Certified Group Psychotherapists.

Ethical issues exist not only related to managed care but also in leading groups in the community where the professional role as occupational therapist can easily become blurred with friend or peer roles. As a therapist, the occupational therapist group leader must make the distinction between "therapy" and "therapeutic." The activities of a working group are inherently therapeu-

Box 10-10
Leadership Education

Occupational therapists who work in various settings need to maintain boundaries and empower their group members to receive services. This may involve resolving conflicts or controversy within the small group or larger institutional setting. Through experiential groups, the student can learn how to influence decision making and power within a group to foster adaptation and group-centered action.

tic. The leader who is a therapist must also assume responsibility for providing therapy by being the group leader, therapist, and professional. As group work is full of choice points, understanding the issues of transference, borrowing from the analytic therapy frame, can help us to make informed choices about what behavior is acceptable on the part of the therapist group leader.

As B. Roth (personal communication, APA Group Psychotherapy List, September 9, 1999) explains, in therapy an asymmetrical power relationship exists between the group and the leader of the group. Further, one cannot act as if meaning does not exist for any actions or anyone's actions. Roth's (personal communication, APA Group Psychotherapy List, September 9, 1999) perspective on the following clinical incident illustrates the benefit of examining the meaning of actions in a group led by a therapist:

A leader agrees for a group to meet in the bedroom of a patient with a broken leg. Roth asks the group therapist, " 'What [member] requests will you deny?' One basic premise of analytic therapy is the transformation from action into words. . . nowhere was the patient's request explored for its meaning. Object constancy also suggests that a meeting take place in your office on a regular and predictable basis. What enactment of transference or conflict is being revealed by the request and the response of taking action? Will you change the time and place again? What fantasies does the patient have? etc., etc. In the analytic community this kind of behavior is viewed as impulsive. . . a transference enactment. . . The so-called boundary exists for the protection of the treatment. It is a frame and violations of the frame are conjointly understood. Actions and requests to change the frame are common in narcissistic patients. . ."

Therapists working in the community would be wise to examine the meanings of member requests and speculate about the ethical choices to be made in light of the asymmetrical relationship between professional role and member role. M. Iosupovici (personal communication, APA Group Psychotherapy List, September 9, 1999) observes, "as treatment is full of choice points, we can only speculate about the choice not taken."

Shifts in models and paradigms of care as well as an emphasis on population-based care require curriculum adjustment. The attention given to the role of occupational therapy in the group treatment of chronic pain is such an area (Weinstein, 1990). As occupational therapists also focus their attention on population-based concerns evolving from social problems, students will find themselves preparing to do functional group work with a constantly changing mix of individuals. More recent population-based programs needing occupational therapy include incarcerated youths with mental health problems (Abras, 1999), substance abusers in self-help groups that support abstinence, families in crisis in family-oriented activities that support cohesion, isolated and violent students in activity groups that aid socialization, and victims of disasters such as floods and earthquakes in task groups that facilitate post-traumatic adjustment. The functional group is suggested as a model for structuring an occupational therapy group process course aimed at student learning of health promotion skills and community-based group leadership (Scott, 1999). See Fig. 10-1.

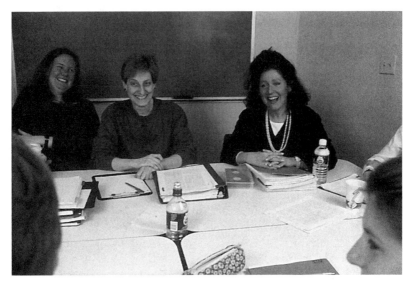

Figure 10-1. Cotherapists in group supervision. (Photograph by Mark Morelli, courtesy of Tufts University, Medford, MA.)

In the supervised clinical experience, the new therapist assumes the role of leader for the first time. This is often a difficult experience, and the support of a supervisor or cotherapist can be invaluable. The supervisor may also provide the feedback necessary to learn from experience. New therapists are frequently impatient with the pace of development in their groups, not realizing that it is difficult for a group to develop mutual concern and caring. The result is too frequent leader intervention and a prolonged dependency of the members upon their leader. An experienced cotherapist or supervisor helps the new therapist to be aware of such problems. In the absence of experienced mentors, novice practitioners can look to peers or other professionals for insight and support.

Review Questions

1. Identify the outcomes of two data-based studies that examine the effects on social interaction.
2. Describe studies that demonstrate the influence of social interaction on the well being of elderly individuals.
3. What outcome variables have been influenced by group format?
4. There are several reports of the effectiveness of group treatment in occupational therapy. Describe these programs and state your rationale.
5. Group treatment has been demonstrated to be cost-effective in occupational therapy. For what types of problems has this been a demonstrated outcome?
6. What issues can we expect to influence the delivery of occupational ther-

apy group programs in the near future? How might these concerns affect curriculum and clinical education experiences?
7. Identify two research questions indicated for further study with concern to a functional approach to group work in occupational therapy.

References

Abras, T. D. (1999). Meeting the mental health needs of adolescents. OT Week May 13, pp. 8–9.

Adelstein, L. A., and Nelson, D. L. (1985). Effects of sharing versus non-sharing on affective meaning in collage activities. Occupational Therapy in Mental Health: A Journal of Psychosocial Practice and Research 5(2): 29–45.

Amini, D. (1999). Patients heal each other. Advance for Occupational Therapy Practitioners May 17: 5,33.

Banning, M. R., and Nelson, D. L. (1987). The effects of activity-elicited humor and group structure on group cohesion and affective responses. American Journal of Occupational Therapy 41(8): 510–514.

Barnes, M. A., and Schwartzberg, S. L. (In press). Activity analysis of group process. Journal of Psychotherapy in Independent Practice.

Barnes, M. A., and Schwartzberg, S. L. (1999). Chapter 10 A Case Study: An Occupational Therapy Approach. In Scott Simon Fehr (Ed.). Introduction to Group Therapy A Practical Guide, pp. 145–146. Binghamton, New York: The Haworth Press.

Borg, B., and Bruce, M. A. (1991). The Group System: The Therapeutic Activity Group in Occupational Therapy. Thorofare, NJ: Slack.

Brinson, M., and Kannenberg, K. R. (1996). Mental Health Service Delivery Guidelines. Bethesda, MD: American Occupational Therapy Association.

Brown, T. (1990). Drama and Occupational Therapy. In J. Creek (ed.), Occupational Therapy and Mental Health, pp. 211–227. New York: Churchill Livingstone.

Bruce, M. A., and Borg, B. (1993). Psychosocial Occupational Therapy Frames of Reference for Intervention, ed. 2. Thorofare, NJ: Slack.

Bruce, M. A. (1988). Occupational therapy in group treatment. In D. W. Scott and N. Katz (eds.), Occupational Therapy in Mental Health Principles in Practice, pp. 116–132. Philadelphia: Taylor & Francis.

Cara, E., and MacRae, A. (1998). Psychosocial Occupational Therapy A Clinical Practice. Albany, NY: Delmar.

Clark, F., Azen, S. P., Zemke, R., Jackson, J., Carlson, M., Mandel, D., Hay, J., Josephson, K., Cherry, B., Hessel, C., Palmer, J., and Lipson, L. (1997). Occupational therapy for independent-living older adults: A randomized controlled trial. Journal of the American Medical Association 278: 1321–1326.

Cole, M. B. (1998). Group Dynamics in Occupational Therapy The Theoretical Basis and Practice Application of Group Treatment, ed. 2. Thorofare, NJ: Slack.

Cole, M. B., and Greene, L. R. (1988). A preference for activity: A comparative study of psychotherapy groups vs. occupational therapy groups for psychotic and borderline inpatients. Occupational Therapy in Mental Health: A Journal of Psychosocial Practice and Research 8(3): 53–67.

Cottrell, R. P. F. (Ed.). (1993). Psychosocial Occupational Therapy Proactive Approaches. Rockville, MD: American Occupational Therapy Association.

DeCarlo, J. J., and Mann, W. C. (1985). The effectiveness of verbal versus activity groups in improving self-perceptions of interpersonal communication skills. American Journal of Occupational Therapy 39(1): 20–27.

Duncombe, L., and Howe, M. C. (1995). Group treatment: Goals, tasks, and economic implications. American Journal of Occupational Therapy 49(3):199–205.

Duncombe, L., and Howe, M. C. (1985). Group work in occupational therapy: A survey of practice. American Journal of Occupational Therapy 39(3): 163–170.

Eklund, M. (1999). Outcome of occupational therapy in a psychiatric day care unit for long-term mentally ill patients. Occupational Therapy in Mental Health 14(4): 21–45.

Eklund, M. (1997). Therapeutic factors in occupational group therapy identified by patients discharged from a psychiatric day centre and their significant others. Occupational Therapy International 4(3): 198–212.

Eklund, M. (1996). Occupational Group Therapy in a Psychiatric Day Care Unit for Long-Term Mentally Ill Patients. Ward Atmosphere, Treatment Process and Outcome. Department of Psychology, Lund University, Lund, Sweden.

Falk-Kessler, J., Momich, C., and Perel, S. (1991). Therapeutic factors in occupational therapy groups. American Journal of Occupational Therapy 45(1): 59–66.

Fleming, M. H. (1991). The therapist with the three-track mind. American Journal of Occupational Therapy 45(11): 1007–1014.

Froehlich, J., and Nelson, D. L. (1986). Affective meanings of life review through activities and discussion. American Journal of Occupational Therapy 40(1): 27–33.

Gauthier, L., Dalziel, S., and Gautheir, S. (1987). The benefits of group occupational therapy for patients with Parkinson's disease. American Journal of Occupational Therapy 41(6): 360–365.

Greene, L. R., and Cole, M. B. (1991). Level and form of psychopathology and the structure of group therapy. International Journal of Group Psychotherapy 41(4): 499–521.

Glass, T. A., Mendes de Leon, C., and Berkman, Lisa F. (1999). Population based study of social and productive activities as predictors of survival among elderly Americans. British Medical Journal 319: 478–483.

Haiman, S. (1990). Selecting group protocols: Recipe or reasoning. In D. Gibson (ed.), Group Protocols: A Psychosocial Compendium, pp. 1–14. Binghamton, NY: The Haworth Press.

Henry, A., Nelson, D., and Duncombe, L. (1984). Choice making in group and individual activity. American Journal of Occupational Therapy 38(4): 245–251.

Howe, M. C., and Schwartzberg, S. L. (1986). A Functional Approach to Group Work in Occupational Therapy. Philadelphia: J. B. Lippincott.

Jackson, J., Carlson, M., Mandel, D., Zemke, R., and Clark, F. (1998). Occupation in lifestyle redesign: The well elderly study occupational therapy program. American Journal of Occupational Therapy 52(5): 326–336.

Kaplan, K. (1986). The directive group: Short-term treatment for psychiatric patients with a minimal level of functioning. American Journal of Occupational Therapy 40(7): 474–481.

Kaplan, K. (1988). Directive Group Therapy Innovative Mental Health Treatment. Thorofare, NJ: Slack.

Kielhofner, G. (1992). Conceptual Foundations of Occupational Therapy. Philadelphia: F. A. Davis.

Kielhofner, G. (1997). Conceptual Foundations of Occupational Therapy, 2nd edition. Philadelphia: F. A. Davis.

Klyczek, J. P., and Mann, W. C. (1986). Therapeutic modality comparisons in day treatment. American Journal of Occupational Therapy 40(9): 606–611.

Knis, L. L. (1995). The play's the THING. OT Week August 31, pp. 18–19.

Kremer, E., Nelson, D., and Duncombe, L. (1984). Effects of selected activities on affective meaning in psychiatric patients. American Journal of Occupational Therapy 38(8): 522–528.

Lee, B., and Nantais, T. (1996). Use of electronic music as an occupational therapy modality in spinal cord injury rehabilitation: An occupational performance model. American Journal of Occupational Therapy 50(5): 362–369.

Locascio, J. (1995). Involving families in psychiatric treatment. OT Week August 24, 1995, pp. 24–25.

Lundgren, C. C., and Persechino, E. L. (1986). Cognitive group: A treatment program for head injured adults. American Journal of Occupational Therapy 40(6): 397–401.

MacKenzie, K. R. (Spring 1999). Professional ethics and the group psychotherapist. The Group Solution. Newsletter of the National Registry of Certified Group Psychotherapists.

Mandel, D. R., Jackson, J. M., Zemke, R., Nelson, L., and Clark, F. A. (1999). Lifestyle Redesign Implementing the Well Elderly Program. Bethesda, MD: American Occupational Therapy Association.

Margolis, R. L., Harrison, S. A., Robinson, H. J., and Jayaram, G. (1996). Occupational therapy task observation scale (OTTOS): A rapid method for rating task group function of psychiatric patients. American Journal of Occupational Therapy 50(5): 380–385.

Marmer, L. (1995). Group treatment works well in stroke recovery. Advance for Occupational Therapists October 2, p. 13.

McDermott, A. A. (1988). The effect of three group formats on group interaction patterns. Occupational Therapy in Mental Health: A Journal of Psychosocial Practice and Research 8(3): 69–89.

Morris, P. A., Andreassi, E., and Lichtenberg, P. (1994). Preparing for community living. OT Week August 25, pp. 20–21.

Nelson, D. L., Peterson, C., Smith, D. A., Boughton, J. A., and Whalen, G. M. (1988). Effects of project versus parallel groups on social interaction and affective responses in senior citizens. American Journal of Occupational Therapy 42(1): 23–29.

Persson, D. (1996). Play and flow in an activity group—A case study of creative occupations with chronic pain patients. Scandinavian Journal of Occupational Therapy 3:33–42.

Polimeni-Walker, I., Wilson, K. G., and Jewers, R. (1992). Reasons for participating in occupational therapy groups: Perceptions of adult psychiatric inpatients and occupational therapists. Canadian Journal of Occupational Therapy 59(5): 240–247.

Posthuma, B. W. (1996). Small Groups in Counseling and Therapy Process and Leadership, ed. 2. Needham Heights, MA: Allyn & Bacon.

Posthuma, B. W. (1989). Small Groups in Therapy Settings: Process and Leadership. Boston: Little, Brown & Company.

Rabinovitch, S. (1999). An experiment with MOHO OT uses model to reverse school's approach to disability. Advance for Occupational Therapy Practitioners August 9, p. 9.

Ross, M. (1987). Group Process Using Therapeutic Activities in Chronic Care. Thorofare, NJ: Slack.

Schulz, C. H. (1994). Helping factors in a peer-developed support group for persons with head injury, Part 2: Survivor interview perspective. American Journal of Occupational Therapy 48(4): 305–309.

Schwartzberg, S. L. and Abeles, J. (1986). Occupational therapy. In L. I. Sederer (ed.), Inpatient Psychiatry, ed.2, pp. 308–323. Baltimore: Williams & Wilkins.

Schwartzberg, S. L. (1999). The use of groups in the rehabilitation of persons with head injury: Reasoning skills employed by the group facilitator. In C. Unsworth Cognitive and Perceptual Dysfunction A clinical Reasoning Approach to Evaluation and Intervention, pp. 455–471. Philadelphia: F. A. Davis.

Schwartzberg, S. L. (1998). Group process. In M. E. Neistadt and Crepeau, E. B. (eds.), Willard and Spackman's Occupational Therapy, ed. 9, pp. 120–131.

Schwartzberg, S. L. (1993). Group process. In H. L. Hopkins and H. D. Smith (eds.), Willard and Spackman's Occupational Therapy, ed. 8, pp. 275–281.

Schwartzberg, S. L. (1994). Helping factors in a peer-developed support group for persons with head injury, Part 1: Participant observer perspective. American Journal of Occupational Therapy 48(4): 297–304.

Schwartzberg, S. L., Howe, M. C., and McDermott, A. (1982). A comparison of three treatment group formats for facilitating social interaction. Occupational Therapy in Mental Health: A Journal of Psychosocial Practice and Research 2(4): 1–16.

Scott, A. H. (1999). Wellness works: Community service health promotion groups led by occupational therapy students. American Journal of Occupational Therapy 53(6): 566–574.

Sorenson, J. R. (1971). Task demands, group interaction and group performance. Sociometry 34: 483–495.

Spitz, H. (Summer 1999). Brief group psychotherapy and managed care: Integration or disconnection? The Group Solution. Newsletter of the National Registry of Certified Group Psychotherapists.

Stahl, C. (1995). Cognition and social competence. Advance for Occupational Therapists, August 7, p.19.

Steffan, J. A. (1990). Productive occupation in small task groups of adults: Synthesis and annotations of the social psychology literature. In A. C. Bundy, N. D. Prendergast, J. A. Steffan, and D. Thorn, Review of Selected Literature on Occupation and Health, pp. 175–281. Rockville, MD: American Occupational Therapy Association.

Steffan, J. A., and Nelson, D. L. (1987). The effects of tool scarcity on group climate and affective meaning within the context of a stenciling activity. American Journal of Occupational Therapy 41(7): 449–453.

Stein, F., and Tallant, B. (1988). Applying the group process to psychiatric occupational therapy, Part 1: Historical and current use. Occupational Therapy in Mental Health 8(3): 9–28.

Tallant, B. (1998). Applying the group process to psychosocial occupational therapy. In F. Stein and S. Cutler (eds.), Psychosocial Occupational Therapy A Holistic Approach, pp. 327–349. San Diego, CA: Singular.

Teasdale, T. W., Christensen, A. L., and Pinner, E. M. (1993). Psychosocial rehabilitation of cranial trauma and stroke patients. Brain Injury 7: 535–542.

Trahey, P. J. (1991). A comparison of the cost-effectiveness of two types of occupational therapy services. American Journal of Occupational Therapy 45(5): 397–400.

Tziner, A., and Eden, D. (1985). Effects of crew composition on crew performance: Does the whole equal the sum of its parts? Journal of Applied Psychology 70: 85–93.

Van Deusen, J., and Harlowe, D. (1987). The efficacy of the ROM dance program for adults with rheumatoid arthritis. American Journal of Occupational Therapy 41(2): 90–95.

Wall, V. D., and Nolan, L. L. (1986). Perceptions of inequity, satisfaction, and conflict in task-oriented groups. Human Relations 39: 1033–1052.

Weinstein, E. (1990). The role of the group in the treatment of chronic pain. Occupational Therapy Practice 1(3): 62–68.

Webster, D. (1988). Patients' perceptions of therapeutic factors in occupational therapy groups. Unpublished master's thesis, Tufts University–Boston School of Occupational Therapy, Medford, MA.

Webster, D., and Schwartzberg, S. L. (1992). Patients' perception of curative factors in occupational therapy groups. Occupational Therapy in Mental Health: A Journal of Psychosocial Practice and Research 12(1): 3–24.

West, W. L. (ed.) (1959). Changing Concepts and Practices in Psychiatric Occupational Therapy. New York: American Occupational Therapy Association.

Index

References in *italics* denote figures; "t" denote tables; "b" denote boxes; and "s" denote sidebars

Actions
  description of, 98–99
  group-centered (*see* Group-centered action)
  purposeful (*see* Purposeful action)
  self-initiated (*see* Self-initiated action)
  spontaneous (*see* Spontaneous action)
Activities of daily living group, 75, 77
Activity groups
  characteristics of, 27t
  description of, 26–27
  goals of, 27
  leader's responsibilities, 30, 30b
  members of, 27–28, 31
  research findings, 246
  theoretical perspective of, 30
  types of, 28–29
Adaptation
  characteristics of, 98t
  definition of, 95s, 96
  description of, 91, 94–95, 96s, 98, 98t
Adaptation Era (1970s to 1990s), occupational therapy groups during
  cost-effectiveness evaluations, 63–64
  description of, 64
  diagnosis-based groups, 61–63
  economic factors, 60
  education programs, 60–61
  medical research advances, 59–60
  roles-based groups, 63
  service delivery models, 63
  setting-based groups, 63
Adaptive response, 96s

Aggressor, 16
Altruism, 25
American Occupational Therapy Association, 55
Archives of Occupational Therapy, 44

Behavior
  group, 6, 11
  imitative, 25
  modeling of, 117–118, 178
  observation of, 127–128
  reality testing of, 118–119
  techniques for assessing, 195, 198
Blocker, 16

Client empowerment, 74
Closed group
  description of, 9–10, 10b
  design stage of, 158–164
  developmental stage of, 210–212
  formation stage of, 185–188
  termination stage of, 229–231
Cohesiveness
  benefits of, 147
  of groups, 9, 19s, 19–20, 26
  member selections and, 147
Coleaders, 129, 205
Collectives, 42–44
Communication skills, of leader
  concreteness, 121
  confrontation, 121–122